MY CHOICE

MY CHOICE

The Ethical Case Against COVID-19
Vaccine Mandates

Dr. Julie Ponesse

The Democracy Fund

2021

The Democracy Fund
61035 Eglinton/Dufferin RO
Toronto, ON
M6E5B2

First edition, December 2021
If you are interested in inviting the author to a live event or
media appearance, please contact us at
https://www.thedemocracyfund.ca/contact

Manufactured in Canada
Cover designed by Lena Yang
Book composed by Karl Hunt
Library and Archives Canada Cataloguing in Publication
Title: My choice : the ethical case against COVID-19 vaccine mandates /
Dr. Julie Ponesse.
Names: Ponesse, Julie, author.
Identifiers: Canadiana 20210382651 | ISBN 9781989555699 (softcover)
Subjects: LCSH: COVID-19 (Disease)—Vaccination—Moral and ethical aspects—
Canada. | LCSH: COVID-19 Pandemic, 2020-—Canada.
Classification: LCC RA644.C67 P66 2021 | DDC 614.4/7—dc23

ISBN 978-1-989555-69-9

ABOUT THE
DEMOCRACY FUND

The Democracy Fund is a Canadian charity dedicated to civil liberties litigation and education, journalism, and humanitarian aid. We are proud to have Dr. Julie Ponesse as our Pandemic Ethics Scholar.

For more information, or to contribute to our cause, please visit www. TheDemocracyFund.ca

For all who keep the flame of hope burning,
even on the darkest days.

CONTENTS

Prologue   ix

Chapter 1: Out of a Job   1

Chapter 2: About Me   8

Chapter 3: Choice and Consequence   15

Chapter 4: Is the Pandemic Response Ethical?   35

Chapter 5: A Way Forward   58

Chapter 6: Do Not Go Gently   81

Appendix 1   94
Appendix 2   98

PROLOGUE

It is undeniable that the COVID-19 pandemic has caused a crisis in health care on a planetary scale. Many thousands of lives have been lost to the virus when existing treatments and public health measures may have made those deaths avoidable or more humane. Our most vulnerable populations, the very old and the very sick, have suffered disproportionately. And apart from the biological toll, COVID-19 continues to deal a massive blow to us socially and psychologically. The UK, for instance, declared a children's mental health crisis months ago, and suicide statistics for children and adolescents have far exceeded their pre-pandemic averages.[1]

1 McMaster Children's Hospital, in Hamilton, Ontario, reported an almost 300% increase in youth suicide attempts between October 2020 and January 2021 compared to the same time period the previous year. McCullough, Kate. "McMaster Children's Hospital reports rise in 'more serious' suicide attempts." (March 18, 2021, https://www.thespec.com/news/hamilton-region/2021/03/18/mcmaster-childrens-hospital-reports-rise-in-more-serious-suicide-attempts.html. Accessed 8 November 2021.)

   In the US, the CDC reported a 24% increase in emergency room mental health visits with children between the ages of 5 and 11. (Leeb RT, Bitsko RH, Radhakrishnan L, Martinez P, Njai R, Holland KM. "Mental Health–Related Emergency Department Visits Among Children Aged <18 Years During the COVID-19 Pandemic — United States. January 1–October 17, 2020." *Morbidity and Mortality Weekly Report,* vol. 69, no. 45, 2020. https://www.cdc.gov/mmwr/volumes/69/wr/mm6945a3.htm?s_cid=mm6945a3_w. Accessed 18 October 2021.

   The American Academy of Pediatrics declared a national emergency in child and adolescent mental health in October 2021 due to soaring rates of mental health challenges among children, adolescents, and their families since the start of the COVID-19 pandemic.https://www.aacap.org/AACAP/zLatest_News/Pediatricians_CAPs_Childrens_Hospitals_Declare_National_Emergency_Childrens_Mental_Health.aspx. Accessed 21 November 2021.

On the therapeutic front, over the last 30 years, more than a third of all vaccine adverse events have been linked to the anti-COVID vaccines.[2] In Canada alone, at the time of writing, over 6000 vaccine recipients have suffered serious side effects, including more than 200 reports with an outcome of death.

But I believe COVID-19 has also triggered a crisis in other institutions we regard as essential to civil, progressive society: academia (most specifically the sciences), journalism, government, and, more broadly, civil discourse. We are living through not just a viral pandemic but a pandemic of coercion and compliance.

I use that last word carefully and deliberately. "To comply" means to "act in accordance with another's will or desire." And this is just what our public health officials are asking of us. Using the media for support, they are demanding we accept their directives and mandates in the absence of compelling evidence and, worse, open debate. As a society, we are all too happy to play along.

We have outsourced our own critical thinking to experts, many of whom have expertise in only the narrowest of areas, or in areas irrelevant to good public policy. Worse, we have turned that act of outsourcing into a civic virtue and in the process we hasten the erosion of our core inalienable rights.

This book is a personal account of my own fight to push back against such erosion, to defend rights I once thought were universally cherished. It is also an examination of the crisis we now face through the lens of ethics and philosophy, disciplines that have formed the bedrock of my professional life. If it provokes

---

2 Over the last 30 years up to August 13, 2021, over 600, 000 VAERS reports of vaccine injuries have been linked to COVID-19 vaccines. As of August 13, 2021, there were a total of 184,886 Serious Adverse Events (SAE) for all vaccines, 80,850 of which were entirely for the COVID-19 vaccines. National Vaccine Information Center. https://medalerts.org/.

the reader to think and question our current circumstances, and to break away from the binary thinking that dominates our public discourse, I will count it as no small victory.

In the *Apology*, Plato quotes Socrates as saying, "the unexamined life is not worth living" (*Apology* 38a). Now, more than ever, we need to abide by that dictum and examine what has happened to our civic life since the pandemic gripped the world.

CHAPTER 1

OUT OF A JOB

The day was warm but drizzly, typical as summers in London, Ontario go. Of course, the importance of the weather had been reduced by COVID restrictions and I was inside, as usual, when the message landed in my inbox with an electronic thud:

Dear Students, Faculty and Staff,

Since the pandemic began, we've worked hard to make the best decisions to protect everyone in the Huron community. We make those decisions based on the best information we have before us.

Right now, we are seeing an alarming rise in the number of COVID-19 cases caused by the Delta variant. At the same time, vaccine supply has increased across Canada—a key line of defense of staving off the virus. Given this information, we've made an important decision alongside Western University and our affiliate partners to keep everyone safe.

As part of a new vaccination policy, all students, staff and faculty will be required to demonstrate proof of vaccination prior to arriving on campus.

Those who cannot provide proof of vaccination will need to complete COVID-19 testing twice weekly.

Western's vaccination and testing centre is open and available to all university community members, meaning you will be able to access testing and Health Canada-approved vaccinations should you need them.

Let me be clear—vaccination is the single most important thing we can do to keep our campus safe. I strongly encourage everyone in our community to get vaccinated, if you are able.

At Huron, we are driven to produce Leaders with Heart, who are aware of and attuned to their communities and their place with them. This is a chance for us to come together and lead by example.

I thank you for your continued patience in this dynamic situation. I look forward to seeing you on campus in September.

Sincerely,
Dr. Barry Craig

Craig is the President of Huron College, the original college of what is now Western University. At its foundation almost 170 years ago, it was a theological school, and it has maintained its focus on philosophy ever since. Huron is where I spent some of my time as an undergraduate, and where I later taught as a professor of ethics and ancient philosophy. I taught students critical thinking and the importance of self-reflection, how to ask good questions and evaluate evidence, how to learn from the past, and why democracy requires civic virtue.

The email landed with a thud, but it wasn't a total surprise. For many months, the academic community across the country had been discussing and debating what an in-person return to classes in the fall of 2021 might look like. Teaching had been exclusively online since the pandemic tightened its grip almost a year and a half earlier. And because of my own focus on medical ethics, I had been thinking and reflecting on the ethical dimension of the pandemic response for some time.

As an ethics professor, I studied the history of vaccines and the mandates that sometimes accompany them. I knew that mandates could happen quickly. So I expected that once COVID became a global phenomenon in early 2020, vaccination was probably going to be the proposed way out. And once vaccination was the proposed way out, it seemed likely that mandates spanning at least the health care and education sectors would follow.

I was further convinced this would happen because governments, over the past few years and especially in the West, have enacted policies under the guise of safety and protection. Its genesis may have been the Patriot Act and its brethren in a post-9/11 world. However it began, we now seem to acquiesce in policies that grant the state a heavy hand. And that trend was made even worse in my own context at the university, where just a few months earlier a new board of governors was appointed, consisting largely of big business figures. A corporatist mindset and a forum for free and honest debate do not often coexist peacefully.

Five days after the directive from Huron was sent, I summarized why I didn't agree with it in an email back to Craig. The details of my objection will fill many subsequent pages of this book but, in short, the foundation of my argument rested on both scientific and ethical grounds. It begins:

> *My primary concern is that the vaccination mandate is not clearly based on evidence-based scientific research, and it violates Canadian human rights law and ethical principles. Where the general health of society is at high risk, the limitations on human rights may be justified, but this case presently cannot be made*

in the situation of COVID-19. This is especially in view of the very low risks of hospitalization and deaths with COVID-19 at this time, the widespread voluntary vaccination and naturally acquired immunity in the population, and the availability of a wide range of counter-active treatments. Please consider what I offer below as an opportunity to rethink Huron's vaccination policy and as an opportunity to engage in a dialogue about these very important issues.

In one of the final paragraphs, I wrote:

In conclusion, the administration of a vaccination is defined as a "medical procedure." The courts have established jurisprudence on informed consent requirements for medical procedures. Furthermore, inquiring into the vaccine status of a student or an employee is a breach of medical privacy (as outlined in the Personal Health Information Protection Act in Ontario, for example), and forcing them to choose between a vaccine and their right to attend school, or take part in certain activities on school grounds, amounts to coercion.

The Aug. 16 email was more than 2,400 words long. It included twenty-four footnotes, most of which point to government sites, official documents, and peer-reviewed research. And I signed it as both an instructor in Huron College's Philosophy Department, and as the Chair of the Ethics and Law Committee of the Canadian Covid Care Alliance (CCCA).

It was met with silence.

The silence from both the administration and my colleagues was both insulting and belittling. In the true spirit of the academy, I had expected—maybe hoped for is more accurate—a response along the lines of "Thank you very much for your concerns. I know this is important to you, especially given that this is one of your areas of study. We value your input."

Even if the decision stood, was it too much to expect something like, "we've weighed all the evidence, we've decided to go in a different way?"

Instead, the responses I was getting, few as they were, were along the lines of, "well, we're just following Health Canada."

When you have a top-down imposition of a mandate on an institution which is supposed to be founded on the idea of free thought and open discourse, and you allow no bottom-up questions or discourse from the members of that community, worries arise for me about the integrity of the process.

In the meantime, I hadn't even started preparing for the fall academic session. Normally professors will order textbooks for their fall classes in June or July but, given the uncertainty over the summer and now facing the possibility that I may not be able to teach at all, I put my setup on hold. It proved to be prescient.

I continued my work with the CCCA, publishing pieces on informed consent, the legal limits of mandates and the uncertainty around vaccine effectiveness. None of this was getting much traction. I sat down with the CCCA's communications team to ponder what we should do next. We asked, "What can we do to bring more attention to this?" My communications with Huron College seemed an obvious place to start.

We decided to record a video with me outlining my stance and thought processes, and the implications for me and for the wider public debate about our COVID response if I did indeed lose my job over my decision.

We recorded the video in the first week of September and published it on the CCCA's Instagram account (and a few other platforms). Despite some platforms removing the video after deeming it "misinformation," it went viral. The Instagram post alone has generated more than 1.1 million views, and it has become a lightning rod for both supporters and detractors. One of the most discussed aspects of the video is the fact I displayed emotion, normally a valuable currency in the social media world.

There is a moment in the latter half of the video (which runs just under five minutes long) where I frame a question for my putative fall class: "This is my first, and potentially my last, lesson of the year." I said it haltingly because tears began to well up. I regained some composure to finish out the video, and as I finished a rush overtook me and I started to cry quietly. One of our communications people said, "oh, I'll edit that out because I don't want you to have to be crying on camera." Then another staffer said, "I think it actually shows the human toll of all of this." We left it in, for better or worse. On the 'worse' end, I struggle with its inclusion because philosophical analysis should be based on reason and not emotion. It also opened me up to accusations of crocodile tears, manufactured to generate sympathy.

Around the same time the video dropped, Huron College announced it was amending its initial vaccination directive (I am not implying any causal connection). It read, in part: "Effective Sept. 7, 2021 all members of our community—including students, employees, and visitors—must provide proof of vaccination or have an exemption, and those with an exemption must be tested for COVID-19 twice weekly. *There is no longer a testing option for those who choose not to be vaccinated.*" (My italics)

I thought it was an odd deletion. If the concern about my vaccine refusal hinges on the danger I could pose as a viral vector, it seems an offer to remove myself physically from the classroom, even the campus as a whole, would be a reasonable measure. We had just lived through more than a year of precedent by teaching online. We already had an administrative apparatus in place to support the strategy; in fact, the class I was scheduled to teach in the fall was Business Ethics, one that I'd taught online many times. Despite my preparatory procrastination, it was practically ready to go either in person or online.

But even though the one allowance that might make it possible for me to teach the fall term had been removed, I still had heard nothing specific to my circumstances from anyone at the college.

Then an email arrived from Huron's Provost and Dean of Arts and Social Sciences, Geoff Read, which made it clear the train had left the station and was picking up speed. He asked pointedly, referring to the Aug. 16 email, "Can we assume from this that you won't comply?" The question didn't even take up one line on my screen.

What I was preparing for mentally was to talk to the Dean and the Chair of my department about possibly revisiting the remote teaching option. But the tenor of the email told me the situation had escalated beyond a simple conversational remedy.

My emailed response was short as well, barely 200 words. From an ethical perspective, I knew it was important for me to be ethically transparent in my thinking (whether that's legally smart, I'll leave for others to decide) so I was clear. I would not comply with any aspect of the mandate. I would not submit proof of vaccination. I would not submit to a rapid test. I would not mask in the classroom.

I waited less than twenty-four hours for the response. On September 16, as I anticipated, Huron College terminated me with cause. I was dismissed for doing exactly what I had been hired to do. I was a professor of ethics, questioning what I view as an unethical demand. You don't have to look hard to see the irony.

CHAPTER 2

ABOUT ME

I could begin this chapter by giving you a rundown of my academic credentials, a career-focused list that would be quite at home on LinkedIn. But I am more than my career, even though my likes, interests, and curiosity bend toward what I do for a living: philosophy and ethics.

The home where I grew up embraced free thought. Both my parents are freethinkers and I'm sure their influence is a major reason I became one, too. Both of them have an unshakeable sense of integrity and live their values every day, even when a different path may appear easier. They are also great at making everything seem special. Big things like Christmas and birthdays, and little things like weekday breakfasts. I think this has had a big impact on my ability to see beauty in surprising places. That they are creative people themselves didn't hurt either.

My outlook was somewhat confirmed in my adult life when I was given a test ostensibly to determine my personality type. Most of you may be familiar with the Myers-Briggs, which is common in the corporate world. While similar in structure, the test I took, the Enneagram, is based on the theory that humans fall into one of nine distinct personality categories.

I fell into category 4: a thoroughgoing individualist. A 4's most basic desire is to be uniquely themselves, to pay less attention to what others think of them, and to derive some of their identity from going against the grain. There were elements of category 5, too (the investigator or observer whose goals are mastery and understanding).

Personality tests like Myers-Briggs and the Enneagram have their fair share of critics and skeptics. But as a descriptive device, the Enneagram helped to explain why I think and act as I do.

It is perhaps unsurprising, then, that I'm drawn to fellow freethinkers. My best friend is the epitome of a freethinker: an artist and writer. She has no advanced degree, yet she is one of the brightest, most creative, and most philosophical people I know. A good lunch date together will involve a mental tussle of open questions, moral quandaries and unsolved problems. That's okay. We embrace them. In fact, we often search them out. We are both quite comfortable living in a vast, open space of grey, as opposed to black and white.

I think that all of these experiences and influences have had a big impact on how I see the world and how I approach things in my life. They have made me very sensitive and also very appreciative of little things, and I've incorporated those sensibilities into my art, especially. These are skills that are indispensable for the artist since they make you more observant and more questioning of subtleties in your environment. They make you slow down or even stop and really look at what you are seeing, and think about why little things matter.

I've been asked more than once about the perceived dichotomy between my passion for art and my interest in academia. But in my eyes, there is no dichotomy: both painting and philosophy are about exploring our existence, creating and examining bold ideas, and interpreting our experiences.

Professionally, my biggest influence was Dennis Hudecki, who still teaches philosophy at Western. He was my first philosophy professor and the first teacher to express real confidence in me as a thinker and a creative person. His confidence was infectious and pushed me beyond a lacklustre elementary and high school education into a deep love of learning in my twenties. Whenever I tackle something new in my life, I can hear him urging me on, expressing amazement, encouragement, and support. Being able to do that for someone else is such an amazing gift. I think we all need someone like that in our lives. Or at least the people who have it are very lucky.

For those still plugged into the LinkedIn mindset, this is who I am professionally:

I received my Ph.D. in ethics and ancient philosophy from the University of Western Ontario. I have a masters in bioethics from the Joint Centre for Bioethics at the University of Toronto and a diploma in ethics from the Kennedy Institute of Ethics at Georgetown University. Until recently I was a professor of ethics with a research specialization in Aristotle's virtue ethics and a background in medical ethics. I have published in the areas of ancient philosophy, ethical theory, and applied ethics. Over the last twenty years, I regularly taught courses in the history of philosophy, political philosophy, ethical theory and applied ethics, including a health care ethics course with a history of medicine component.

I am well versed in the fundamental principles of contemporary bioethics and in the balancing of these in the context of public health, including an understanding of the thresholds that must be met in order to justify vaccination mandates, which limit personal rights and freedoms for the sake of the collective good. I have expertise in the ethical dimensions of voluntary informed consent in the context of health care, and of international documents like the Nuremberg Code and the Universal Declaration on Bioethics and Human Rights, which aim to protect people from medical experimentation.

And I'm also an attentive student of the history of medicine, which offers a number of examples of the corruption of regulatory systems as well as the human costs of employing profit incentives in pharmaceutical decision-making.

I didn't imagine there would be a life for me outside of academia, or that there would need to be. Now I can hardly imagine still being there. Seeing it from the outside gives you a different perspective.

Throughout my academic life, I had a feeling just above the subconscious level that I was writing, experiencing, living someone else's story. The discipline and culture never felt like a perfect fit for me. There were parts that I liked: the history of thought, the intellectual freedom to explore all the 'nooks and crannies' of an idea, the performance art that is lecturing, helping students to develop an appetite for learning and a healthy sense of curiosity about the world around them.

But in other ways, I was always a bit of a misfit. Might I have fit better forty years ago or 500 years ago, or even 2,500 years ago?

Some have called me an "academic pariah" which, far from a pejorative, prompts me to think of Socrates and how he was portrayed 2,500 years ago in Plato's dialogue, *Meno*.

In the dialogue, Meno compares Socrates to a torpedo fish (an archaic term for an electric ray) which shocks or numbs its prey into silence by simply asking questions (in this case, about virtue). Socrates' response is worth noting: "As for me, if the torpedo is torpid itself while causing others to be torpid, I am like it, but not otherwise. For it is not from any sureness in myself that I cause others to doubt: it is from being in more doubt than anyone else that I cause doubt in others." (*Meno* 80c-d)

11

My questioning of authority and received wisdom is not meant as a sign of personal certainty; it's an expression of the doubt I have about what I'm being told is true. I firmly believe nobody owns the truth, particularly concerning the current pandemic. Yet public officials and a significant portion of the general population act as if all questions related to COVID have been answered. And so questioners, me included, are cast out today in much the same way that people in Plato's Greece avoided, and ultimately persecuted, Socrates.

Today we treat words like *science* and *expert* as synonyms for perfection. And we idolize those concepts. I'm not sure we know what they mean, but we idolize them nonetheless. And if you're on the so-called side of science and the experts, you are not only on the right side intellectually, but you are virtuous, you are morally good, you are a good citizen, you are a good democratic participant. And if you are not on the side of the scientists and the experts (whoever has decided what that means), then not only are you wrong but you're shut down, and you're excluded, and your voice no longer matters.

Beyond a nagging sense of fit or belonging, I've grown to think there is something a bit ironic, even disingenuous, about *teaching* ethics; the discipline is really something that needs to be lived, tried, modelled in the real world.

In a way, that feeling has been the genesis of this book. For many months now, I have lived (imperfectly, no doubt) many of the theoretical constructs of ethical philosophy. For many months now, I have been both subject and observer in a live laboratory, testing the tenets of disciplines that in some cases stretch back millennia.

One of the most surprising and disheartening facets of living this experiment has been an assessment of the role of social ostracization today. For more than a decade, social media has dominated our metrics of fame, attention, even personal worth. As a social species, humans have always needed to belong. But the digital world has amplified the need and made it ubiquitous.

I often wonder why it is so important to others to just get along, to dissolve into the group. Maybe we crave belonging to a group because it gives us a sense of identity that is somehow easier to come by than getting it from ourselves. Individualism takes more work. It requires more self-knowledge ("know thyself," a quotation that Dioegenes Laertius attributed to Thales of Miletus, who predates Plato by 200 years), perhaps more intellectual multi-tasking. Offloading these tasks to the group not only reduces mental workload but also displaces responsibility. "If I didn't come up with it myself, then I'm not responsible if things go wrong."

Many people I encounter are quite shocked that I am willing to take such an unpopular public stand. What that says to me is that belonging, not being cast out by the tribe, is very high on their list of values. For me, it just isn't. Chalk it up to being a Type 4, or to Socrates the torpedo fish. The fact is, feeling like I am in step with the tribe usually *unsettles* me. It makes me question whether the belief I have in common with the tribe is really my belief. I am skeptical, I guess, of conforming.

Plato's student, Aristotle, had something to say about this. In his *Nicomachean Ethics,* he posits reputation as one possible path to happiness. A common Greek idea was that a good reputation among your peers is the way to the best life; a bad reputation leads to a lonely, empty life. That may be true, as far as it goes, but as maintained by Aristotle, such an approach is no recipe for a happy, flourishing life. Reputation is fleeting, often beyond personal control: it is outside oneself.

Reputation, in this sense, sits opposite morality, which is about character, the essence of who you are. You can't choose what reputation you have among others. But you absolutely can choose to act morally, in defiance of all that's around you. I think my freethinking family and friends would applaud that last sentence.

CHAPTER 3

CHOICE AND CONSEQUENCE

The two decisions made in September, my decision to resist the vaccination mandate, and the college's decision to fire me with cause, have been among the most pivotal of my life. Assessing how they have affected me has been an evolutionary process. They've hurt me personally, professionally, and emotionally. But they've helped me too. In this chapter, I want to explore the aftermath of those decisions and how it has shaped me as both a person and a citizen.

The college's termination letter stated I was being fired not just because of my unwillingness to cooperate with the mandate to vaccinate, but because I was spreading disinformation and using the issue for personal promotion. The disinformation was connected to two issues: one, my doubts about the medical and ethical effectiveness of the COVID response and, two, my assertion at the time of the video that Huron College had already terminated me.

The latter may have been an error on my part, although I took their initial quick response stating I was suspended immediately as a signal, I was now headed down a one-way street. The ensuing radio silence from the college also struck me as entirely antithetical to the soul of the academy. I was being fired for doubting on both scientific and ethical grounds the legitimacy of the vaccine mandate and attendant lockdown measures. No discussion, no debate, no plan to compromise at all.

The days immediately following the termination letter remain a whirlwind in my mind. The video, already viral, was given rocket fuel. Its popularity is wholly ironic. In my art career, I'm always asking friends and fellow artists, "How do you get traction on social media? What kind of posts do you have?" I am the least savvy person when it comes to the vagaries of viral social content. Yet here the response was beyond anything I ever anticipated.

Corporate media began saturating my phone and inbox with interview requests. Reporters were trying to connect on an hourly basis. They sugar-coated their intentions to lure me in, and then wrote articles affirming the narrative that I'm a misguided (or worse, malicious) "anti-vaxxer" spreading misinformation.

Invitations to speak to various groups came in fast and furious. All that against a backdrop of growing social media reaction, both positive and negative.

The negative was to be expected. Online attacks are the lifeblood of platforms like Twitter and my circumstances were ideal for a pile-on. Typical were tweets like this: "We are fighting a malignant, highly contagious virus and we need to stand together to fight COVID. Your BS is self-serving and malicious. You are anti-Canadian."

But the reaction of many of my colleagues, those I worked with at Huron and Western, as well as those in the larger academic community, have been the most biting and in some ways the hardest to understand. They were delivered both on and off social media.

Jacob Shelley, a Western law professor and director of the university's Health Ethics, Law & Policy Lab, has been among my harshest critics on digital platforms. Twitter is his preferred venue, where he has called me, among other things, "disingenuous and deceitful." Although he has responded to some of my statements with factual takedowns, including a multi-tweet thread, most of his tweets have been decidedly *ad hominem*:

> She's a grifter. I have responded to @DrJuliePonesse and she won't engage because she prefers to lie and build her career. She's chosen to exploit this opportunity . . . She's only lauded amongst conspirators.

Reacting to an announcement of my appearance in mid-November at a town hall with journalist John Stossel (hosted by Ezra Levant and Dr. Charles McVety of Canada Christian College, both controversial figures to be sure), Shelley tweeted:

> Would someone that really taught critical thinking be involved with Charles McVety? Forget Ezra for the moment—McVety is truly a terrible person. How does that align with what you taught @DrJuliePonesse? Guessing you won't respond, just more tears about your 'suffering.'

Other colleagues were similarly focused on attacking me personally. James Crimmins, a political theory professor at Huron, tweeted:

> Shameful disregard for the facts. The Socratic method is designed to eliminate what is manifestly false, not merely to raise questions. The sophistry pedaled (sic) here is dishonest, and raises the question what else of dubious merit this professor teaches.

He followed up later, adding:

The professor does not teach medical ethics and nor does she have credentials in this area. That she has aligned herself with people all too willing to promote the untried drug Ivermectin confirms her questionable moral compass.

The *Toronto Star* solicited this take from Arthur Caplan, the founding director of the Division of Medical Ethics at New York University Langone Medical Center: "People spend a little more time listening to ethics professors about ethics," he said. "I've been working on vaccines for nine years, and I wouldn't pass her in my ethics class."

But among the hardest blows were the reactions of Anthony Skelton, a Western professor specializing in moral philosophy and its history. Anthony and I have been on friendly terms in the past, on and off campus, and our history together goes back to my time as a masters student at the University of Toronto. After the viral video appeared, he didn't contact me. But he did tweet:

> Shame on Julie Ponesse. This is the anti-thesis of the Socratic mission: to live the examined life. Ponesse's remarks about COVID-19 vaccines and vaccine mandates rest on moral and factual errors.

We haven't talked since.

While I knew those particular critics, most of the attacks on me have come anonymously, at best behind an avatar and only in text form. That doesn't mean they don't carry emotional weight. They aren't necessarily less harmful just because they're not face-to-face. The relative anonymity may make the invective easier to hurl—it may make the intensity easier to ratchet upward—but I think all that does is impose a greater burden on the aggressor to be responsible with their insults and accusations.

Online attacks that belittle my intelligence and question my virtue have the potential to take their toll. They're emblematic of what I see as a mob culture that embraces bullying behaviour as its enforcement mechanism. We see this behaviour in elementary school, in the playground, but social media has revealed many of us never outgrow it, which is incredibly sad and disturbing.

The irony is not lost on me: many of my critics are educated in ethics and morals yet appear to cast aside the restraint that should come with such an education. Of course, they say the same about me, that my training as an ethicist should make me realize the error of my stance.

But let us ask: why are people who have spent entire careers steeped in ethics unable or unwilling to have a respectful and probing discussion about the ethical dimensions of the issues before us? Why does the dialogue so quickly degenerate?

I realize I'm an easy target because I put a video out into the world in which I clearly take a strong counter-narrative position, and then break down emotionally near the end. You couldn't be more vulnerable than that. They haven't done that. Most are just firing shots from behind an anonymous stone wall.

There is one person at Western who has stood by me: my first philosophy professor, Dennis Hudecki, who I mentioned in the previous chapter. His was the very first class of my very first year at university. After a lackluster and uninspiring elementary and high school education, walking into his class felt like a breath of fresh air. He constantly asked for our thoughts on current events and he was obviously genuinely interested in our answers. As a teacher, he had enormous passion for questioning and critical thinking and history and imagination and exploration. He, more than anyone else, shaped my academic career and who I became (and tried to become) as a professor.

He is standing by through all of this, quietly, and I know he discusses pandemic ethics, including the details of my circumstances in his classes. We don't talk often but his presence in the background is still a source of strength to me. Louis Charland, a longtime member of the Philosophy and Health Sciences Departments at Western, was also a source of rich and supportive discussion in the early days of my thinking about these issues. Unfortunately, and devastatingly, Louis died suddenly from a heart attack in May 2021.

Apart from Hudecki, most of the Western University community is now largely an alien landscape. I knew once I made my decision, I would never work there again. This is a place that holds a lot of meaning for me. I was an undergraduate there; I earned my PhD there. Many beloved professors who taught me and who I worked closely with are still there.

The silence from colleagues has been eerie. I have heard nothing from any of my fellow professors at Huron. Not "I don't agree with you, but wow this must be hard." Or even "I disagree with you and I'd like to discuss it with you." The response has been simply distancing and dismissal.

It is striking to me that the word *professor* is related to the Latin for *declare openly, testify voluntarily, acknowledge*, and *take a vow*. A professor isn't someone who just reads, researches, publishes, runs the occasional lecture or seminar, but someone who is willing to declare publicly her findings and opinions, discuss them with others, and when required live these principles even when doing so is inconvenient, or worse, comes with the greatest risks.

Socrates, Plato's mentor, and, according to many, the first true professor of philosophy, didn't write anything (as far as we know). He went around Athens engaging people in conversation, asking hard questions, and not shying away from uncomfortable topics.

He didn't stop until the truth came out. Socrates was hardly an expert; in fact, he is famous for having professed his ignorance: whereas I, as I do not know anything, do not think I do either (*Apology* 21d). And yet he was better at getting at the truth than anyone, just by asking questions. This is a tough but worthwhile goal. It isn't clear Canada of the twenty-first century would make room for Socrates. It isn't clear we wouldn't accuse and convict him, as the Athenians did.

In terms of relationship losses, I think COVID-19 and my public comments about it have been, in many ways, a test of the strength of existing relationships. Some relationships, or people, didn't pass the test. The recent situation has shown who they really were, or maybe who I really was. We've already covered the many philosophy colleagues who have abandoned, ignored, or publicly shamed me, calling me ignorant, blind, arrogant, and even selfish. In terms of my art career, I lost relationships with customers and some existing commission contracts. I also lost an important relationship with a local gallery owner, someone I had been rather close to and with whom I have had very thoughtful, deep conversations over the last couple of years.

The bad comments hurt. *Of course* they do. I haven't been able to shake "grifter" since I first saw the slur. And it perplexes me why people like my former professional colleagues keep coming after me. But I plod along. To try to capture the feeling in an image as accurately as possible, it feels a bit like being poked by little arrows while trying to climb up a steep mountain face. Yes, the words hurt as arrows might. And being at the leading edge can be exhausting. Why some want to keep going, I don't know. I guess for me the little pains from the arrows pale by comparison to the thought of what we might lose if we don't reach the summit, or if we give up trying.

I want to be clear that I didn't make my decision knowing I had a soft place to land. I knew the risks and costs, and knew some would be deeply personal. But I did it anyway because it was clear this was the only choice that made sense—moral and personal sense.

But it would be fair to say that some relationships have been strengthened, too. While I have been surprised by many of the people who have abandoned and shamed me, I have also found new power and new avenues for exploration within existing relationships and have also forged new bonds with new people that would never have happened without the whirlwind of the past few months.

I have found support and deep friendship in surprising places. People who I thought had views quite different from my own have either expressed their support for my position or just support for my right to express them. My relationship with my closest friend has grown immensely, largely because we have found a way to approach even the most delicate of subjects with honesty, thoughtfulness and grace.

And the cliché rings true for me: as one door closes, another opens. I am writing and speaking and talking with interesting people now more than ever. People who are engaged and truly concerned about issues that matter. Freedom. Responsibility. Safety. Health in all its forms, physical, mental, and emotional.

Several months before the confrontation with Huron College reached its peak, I became involved with the Canadian Covid Care Alliance. It seems some staff working for the alliance had seen a YouTube video I posted in the spring of 2021, along with a follow-up video interview I did with Maxime Bernier, the leader of the People's Party of Canada. Bernier was gearing up for the predicted fall federal election and was keen to make the ethics of Canada's COVID response an election issue.

The CCCA contacted me and said, "We think you'd be a good fit. Do you want to come and join our group?" The group was made up of doctors and scientists in the fields of health care and biology (including immunologists, virologists, toxicologists, pathologists and epidemiologists), along with people who had experience with law and ethics. Many of these people are tenured or even full professors at top Canadian universities. Collectively, those in the alliance say they "have serious concerns with respect to the management of the COVID-19 pandemic in this country." My father is a family doctor in a small town in Ontario and I grew up with medicine as part of my life. The science is not foreign to me. The CCCA sounded like a place where my voice could be heard, my expertise appreciated, and where working together toward a common set of goals could produce results. The more I became involved, the more I realized I was surrounded by bright, dedicated people, and that we just might make a difference.

My work with the CCCA has put me firmly in the public spotlight, and the requests for appearances and media interviews have mushroomed since I was fired by the university. The increased exposure has also led to another role for me in the debate over our approach to COVID: I joined The Democracy Fund. It is a not-for-profit Canadian civil liberties organization with a strong focus on COVID-related public health measures that have had an impact on our freedom and civil rights. My role focuses on education and analysis around pandemic ethics, in both a strictly academic sense and also in the realm of public policy.

Ezra Levant has been the spearhead of The Democracy Fund, and I'm acutely aware of the fact he is a socio-political lightning rod in this country. I have been challenged by many over my association with the charity and, by extension, Levant. Why would I link up with someone so polarizing and controversial, the focus of hate for so many Canadians? It's an easy answer, one that has its roots in classical philosophy.

I would never refrain from associating with someone, professionally or personally, just because other people thought poorly of that person. That's a personal principle which I first learned reading what Aristotle had to say in the *Ethics* (which I'll say more about in the following chapter). In its volumes, Aristotle ponders the essence of the good. Many of his contemporaries believed the good to be synonymous with honour and public reputation. He thought that was a weak foundation, essentially relegating goodness to what others think of you. Its closest contemporary analogue is celebrity.

Celebrity is vacuous. The concept has less to do with who you are as a person, and more to do with the person making the evaluation. It is subject to fads and temporal whims, and to politically driven narratives. It is not a reflection of you, it's a reflection of what's going on inside somebody else.

So I know what's said about these people and their groups, Ezra Levant, Rebel, Maxime Bernier, PPC, The Democracy Fund. Rebel, for instance, is flashy. No doubt about it. When you visit the site, it tries to grab you, everything from the colours to the graphics to the nature of the headlines is going for your eyeballs. It doesn't mean everything that's there is untrue or over-the-top salacious. Or if even some of it is, how is it different from many other corporate media outlets? Every news agency we can name is vying for your attention by using the same bag of tricks. Attention is currency, so they do what they can to get noticed. The point is, we place an awful lot of value in the public perception of a person or entity, and the picture of that person or entity that gets presented to the world, and which is built up by the combined forces of the media and the public over time often, very often distorts reality.

My experience has been one-to-one, and I can tell you getting to know these people and groups on an even slightly deeper level has been revelatory. And quite unlike their public perception. It has reinforced Aristotle's skepticism of placing too much stock in public perceptions of reputation: take all of it with a grain of salt.

I use the layers-of-an-onion analogy. There's a lot of effort put into building a caricature of a thing now, helped along by media, social and otherwise. I'm learning that the real thing is often very loosely connected to that caricature and also that, like the layers of an onion, people are complex in ways a superficial glimpse can never reveal. I personally wouldn't take as a guide what other people think about a journalist or an academic or a news agency. I'd want to look into it myself first. If I want to be associated with that group because I think they're doing good work, then I'm going to do it regardless of what people think. I'm going to try to peel back those layers to get to the heart of what that person really is.

Having said that, I don't think my style is to be like Rebel. There's still a lot of the reserved academic in me. I try to be more dispassionate and analytical, and I can afford to be because that's both my pedigree and the role I've chosen to play in the aftermath of my formal academic career.

The basic truth underlying the experiences I've had meeting these more prominent public figures and their associates is this: I've been awakened to a determined group of Canadians who think deeply about issues such as freedom and responsibility the same way I do, and who do it never having entered a faculty lounge or defended a doctoral thesis. Many more are fighting an internal battle to stay sane in the face of increasingly irrational and untrustworthy actions done in the name of public safety.

Many people from all over the world have written to me, easily more than 2,000 since Huron fired me. Most of them say a variant of, "I'm so sorry for what you went through." I say to them (when I've had the ability to write back), "I really appreciate that. Thank you. And as well-meaning as those comments are, and I greatly appreciate them, in some sense they don't resonate with me because that is not the essence of my sadness. Just to be clear, I'm not upset about my personal situation. I'm devastated that we've gotten to this place in Canada where you can be dismissed so easily, cast aside so easily, for challenging, for questioning."

The tears I cried in that September video weren't crocodile tears, and they certainly weren't tears of self-pity. They were the tears of a mother who harbours a growing sense of dread thinking about what the world is going to be like for her and her child. That is the wave that throws you down and rolls over you in an endless torrent, so much that it's almost too hard to hold in your head all at once. It's a wave that strips you of reason and intellect and leaves you with only the tatters of your emotions to make sense of the world. That is not enough.

So many respondents have been hit by the same wave. So many write the same words: "When I saw your tears, I felt my own." So many people all over the world are going through the same thing.

Something else I hear more lately: "Oh, you're such a hero." Really? I'm a hero for deciding I don't want to be forced to put something in my body? I'm a hero for not wanting to be a victim of a state-mandated assault in some sense? Far from heroism, I think it says more about where we are than about who I am as a person. The unique thing about me as a person is that I just care so little about what other people think, and that's rare. That's anomalous. That's what allows me to weather all of this. But maybe it *is* heroism. If so, I cannot get out of my mind the idea that our culture never should have put someone in a position where such an action deserves any kind of *heroic* label.

That touches on one of my motivations for doing this at all. Showing people that it's possible and that, through it all, you're still standing. That's important. People need to feel that there is security in numbers, that there's a place to land if they have to fall at all. Some have even noted my own circumstance and said, "Well, you got a better job out of this than the one that you had, so I guess that wasn't so bad."

There is truth to that sentiment. I'd never have guessed when I created the September video that it would go viral. Now most of the statements I put out (whether video or text) touch people around the world. I joked earlier about the trouble I had getting any kind of public notice of my paintings. Now I'll get a question from a Swiss news outlet asking if it's OK to translate a recent speech I gave into German. It's completely surreal and wonderful at once.

And as my messages have started reaching a broader audience (both geographically and demographically) I've sensed a kind of untethering of ideas from the institution they're normally associated with. There is a world beyond the Richmond Street gates of Western University where people think and talk about interesting and provocative ideas all the time. Sometimes more effectively than in any academic setting. The conversations I've had with thinkers like Julius Ruechel (an author who doesn't have a graduate degree, as far as I know) are more interesting than most any I had within the confines of the academy. We must be careful about our assumptions: they can quickly turn to elitism and over-specialization, and portray people outside our narrow band of experience as having no value in public discourse.

I'm still in touch with other academics who tell me they rarely, if ever, have such stimulating and engaging conversations. Not even a free-ish exchange of ideas. If they have them at all, they have to work very hard for them. They'll say things like, "Well, my Chair and I have a workable relationship, and I sometimes corner colleagues and try to engage them in conversation." Which is quite sad and likely an indication of how institutionalized bullying has deeply penetrated the academy. When having "proper" thoughts is considered more desirable than thinking itself, the soul of academic life is in danger.

* * *

I've grown increasingly disheartened about the breakdown of open communication in our society. Our nation is supposed to be a leader in terms of democracy and citizen participation, and our academic institutions are supposed to be the fulcrum of that democracy. They're supposed to be the place where we can exchange ideas and ask questions freely and without fear of censure and with support. That doesn't mean that everybody within those institutions will always agree with one another. That is an impossible, and I think misguided, ideal. But it does mean, in my mind, that we approach each other, especially those with whom you disagree, with curiosity and openness and acceptance. And that when you hear something from another person that you don't understand or you don't necessarily agree with, that's an invitation not to shut them down but to ask more questions or, if desired, push back with counter-arguments and evidence, and not character attacks. "Tell me why you think this? Show me some evidence. Explain to me why you feel so strongly about it." But we're seeing this ideal form of intellectual engagement breaking down in our universities and, in fact, all sectors of society. And the more it breaks down, the weaker our foothold on democracy becomes, a foothold that may be very hard to restore.

This devolution has been happening slowly and insidiously for quite sometime. It's very clear within some disciplines and within departments and even entire schools at universities that certain lines of questioning are accepted and certain lines are not.

When we're critically examining information about COVID-19 and pandemic response policies, issues that are highly based on data and information, it's vitally important how we handle that information. We must be careful not to reject certain kinds of data without due cause. Because when we do that, and we've seen it happen throughout the history of science and the history of education, we close off possibilities for further exploration and further development. And we do ourselves a great disservice. For, as we have often learned the hard way, "History doesn't repeat itself, but it often rhymes."

I haven't spent very much time on the administrative side of the table during my university career but I perceive a growing trend with many administrators, who now see their role as more in line with the CEO of a corporation than as the leader of a group of thinkers and learners. Now, this isn't to say all corporations are bad or misguided or ultimately do not serve humanity. But I believe when you put on such a hat you start thinking in terms of the sanctity of the bottom line, and money and public perception both grow in importance. Maybe they eclipse the subjects that you're teaching. And more fundamentally than that, a corporate outlook torques the ways you allow people within your institution to communicate with one another, to raise ideas and to affect change. Rarely for the better.

That is why I'm heartened that I no longer have such constraints. But even though my freedom to think and the resulting reach of my thoughts and statements have blossomed in the past few months, there has been a psychological cost. I feel a growing pressure to be perfect in everything I say and do because I know all eyes are on me now.

I know critics are waiting in the shadows, ready to pounce on every misstep and gaffe I make. They'll employ the illogical but often effective tactic of "See, she's wrong about this, therefore, she's wrong about everything." But it's not just a fear of slipping up in front of haters. It's a fear of letting down an audience that is now counting on you to fix our broken system, people who are rooting for you because they care about their lives and they need solutions. But they can't affect change on their own. If you don't do a good enough job, you feel like you've failed them.

That is enormous pressure, not as easy to ignore as the harsh criticisms coming from the other side. While Aristotle's *Ethics* should apply in both instances, the sense of letting down an ally is a more powerful motivator than the invective of a perceived enemy.

I cope with the pressure by realizing the magnitude of the crisis in front of us and by trying to imagine a post-crisis world where liberal values and a return to a more liberal approach to public health prevails.

There is, quite undeniably, a crisis in health care. Lives have been lost to COVID-19 when existing early outpatient pharmaceuticals may have made deaths avoidable or easier; children especially have suffered from the lockdown measures (the UK, as mentioned, declared a children's mental health crisis months ago); and more than a third of all vaccine adverse events over the last 30 years have been linked to the set of COVID-19 vaccines.[3]

---

3   Rose, Jessica. "A report on the US Vaccine Adverse Events Reporting System (VAERS) of the COVID-19 messenger ribonucleic acid (mRNA) biologicals." *Science, Public Health Policy & the Law*, vol. 2, 2021.

But I believe we also have a crisis in science, academia, journalism, government, and civil discourse. We are living through not just a viral pandemic, but a pandemic of coercion and compliance. I say "compliance" because "to comply" means to "act in accordance with another's will or desire." And this is just what our public health officials are asking of us. Using the media for support, they are demanding that we accept their directives and mandates in the absence of evidence and open debate. As a society, we are all too happy to play along. We have turned the outsourcing of our own critical thinking into a civic virtue and, in the process, we are hastening the erosion of our core inalienable rights.

Quite apart from the circumstances of my own break from academia, I can't see myself ever returning. Not in a formal sense, at least.

I had an odd experience recently, something many others likely go through when they change careers or retire. I was trying to clean up my computer because the hard drive was maxing out its storage capacity. Some of the bulkiest items on the drive are PowerPoint presentations for big, three-hour classes I used to teach. I went through the process of pondering, "will I need that again? I can't throw it out, I may use it next time . . ." Until I realized, no. I'm not ever going to need to teach in that way again.

That was a moment of confrontation with a kind of reality. And it was an acceptance, a decision to act. Even though there's a microscopic chance I'll need those PowerPoints again, it was more important to proceed with the purge, the catharsis, the cleaning of the slate.

If I ever have to rebuild those slides, it will be a for a very good reason. But, honestly, I don't see myself returning to the academy. I feel the loss of the community and I feel betrayal from people within the community. I don't think I'll ever earn the respect of those people again. And it's very hard to imagine a day when my respect for them will return in a robust way. Beyond the trust and respect issues, being a professor is not what I always wanted to do, not in the formal sense of the role. I've always wanted to think deeply about important things. I always found ethics tremendously interesting and compelling. And at the onset of my teaching career, I found the dialogue in the classroom with students interesting and helping them to explore ideas was rewarding. But those moments have proven fleeting, and both those moments and the skills needed to tease them out are transferable. They don't need to happen only within the university walls, and increasingly they're happening less and less within those walls. So, I have found the last few years of teaching, with a few exceptions, to be quite mind-numbing. The routine of it all sapped the joy; the loss of camaraderie made it feel empty; the indifference of the more recent student cohorts made it feel pointless. If nobody cares what I have to say, why speak at all?

I was at a meeting the other day and a thought occurred to me that I put up for discussion: "When you're within academia, you feel a bit like the world falls off at its edge. If you leave it, it's almost like leaving an intellectual cult-like culture." But my experience of leaving has not been that. It was more like a breath of fresh air, the same sensation I had when I took my first university philosophy class with Dennis Hudecki after years of academic suffocation. It's been made real to me of late that interesting ideas don't happen only in academic journals or at universities. There are smart people who are thinking about interesting things and engaged in interesting ideas and questions all over the place. And for me, it feels quite freeing. And if I'm going to do work like this, I'm really happy to be doing it in a place where the ideas are not just confined to academic journals, publications that reach a tiny, narrow audience, and are not just tools for promotion and tenure rather than enlightenment or debate fodder.

It makes me only a little sad that I lost my job for doing something I still have a passion for, that is supposed to be very much within the confines of our legal system and our bioethical principles. But am I doing the right thing?

Sometimes you can't answer that in the heat of battle. You must wait until the dust settles to examine your actions and their effects honestly. But people still ask: "Well, how do you feel about things, moving forward?" I usually answer this way: you know you've done the right thing when you have a peaceful conscience, when you can sleep at night, when you don't have that nagging feeling that there was some stone left unturned or something better or more that you ought to have done.

I don't have that nagging feeling. I do have a measure of peace. That doesn't mean that there is not a set of unpleasant consequences, including really harsh feedback from colleagues, media stories, the social fallout, and all of that. But in the end, we come back to Aristotle. Those negatives don't really matter because they're about reputation. They aren't really about me and my core.

Honesty demands I admit this much: if all of this went away, I'd be quite happy. My official title at The Democracy Fund is Pandemic Ethics Scholar. That's not transferable. As soon as the pandemic goes away, there's no more pandemic ethics, and there's no more position. Yet if I woke up tomorrow and the headlines blared, "Pandemic over," I would think, "Okay, excellent. I can go back to a simpler life." I would like all of this to go away so I can go upstairs and play with my daughter and read her books and soak in every moment as she grows up. I don't want to be in this arena a moment longer than I need to be. I see the comments people make on YouTube or other social media platforms, pleas like, "She should be our health minister. She should run for prime minister." I don't want any of that. I believe to my core that it's important that we do it right when it comes to this issue and its attendant problems. And I know how critical it is for Canadians to put the right people in the right positions. But these are not personal goals of mine.

I just want to help to get Canada back on some better footing so that my daughter and every other child in our country can have a better life.

CHAPTER 4

IS THE PANDEMIC RESPONSE ETHICAL?

This chapter's signature question has occupied my thoughts almost since the onset of COVID-19, and (without boasting) I'd say I'm well prepared to address it. After all, the question goes to the heart of my intellectual life. I've been trained and educated to answer it, and questions like it, or at least to begin the tough task of parsing some of the key issues, and thinking about how we might move through them.

The shorthand version of my answer is this: most of the measures employed to counter the pandemic aren't prompted or supported by the data, and those measures carry grave physical, political, and ethical consequences. We use a faulty testing system to generate case numbers; we apply the same measures to all people (even though we know that COVID-19 poses different risks to different people of different ages); we ignore existing, effective treatment options; we mandate investigational vaccines under the false notions that there are no effective alternatives and that these vaccines are safe; and then we continue to hold the narrative even as data emerge which blatantly undermines it.

Beneath the overarching question lie some others that I'll tackle on their own merits: what are the relevant ethical principles we need to consider? Autonomy, nonmaleficence, beneficence, justice—all are in play in this assessment. What conditions justify vaccine mandates? Do the circumstances we face now meet those conditions? Are we able to use historical precedent, our experiences with previous pandemics and mass vaccination campaigns, to inform our approach in the twenty-first century? What role do experts play in determining what measures are ethical? And we need also to ask, "what *is* an expert when it comes to COVID-19 policy?"

The ethics of the global COVID-19 response are largely the ethics of public health. At its core, public health is concerned with promoting and protecting the health of populations. Mandates aimed at protecting public health are ethically justified to the extent that they create a favorable risk/benefit ratio with respect to the public good and that they are appropriately balanced, with limitations on personal autonomy. Public health mandates often involve, even require, coordinated action on the part of regulatory bodies and governments. But how and to what ends these entities work together to create and support vaccination mandates affects, whether or not those mandates are justified.

There are two main aspects of vaccination mandates that pose unique ethical challenges and both require careful attention: balancing the collective good with limitations on personal autonomy, and the authority of the state or private entities to implement measures that protect public health.

The challenges prompt some important questions: how much can we ask people to sacrifice in order to achieve public health, and what threshold must be met in order to justify limitations on our private choices? These questions touch on a well-worn debate in public health ethics between reductionists and anti-reductionists, and it isn't necessary to rehearse the specifics of that debate here.

What is important to understand is that public health ethics is a balancing act. It is almost inevitable that public health policies will come at the cost of some personal rights and freedoms. The challenge is to determine when those limitations are justified and when they go too far.

The word *autonomy*, from the Greek words for "self" and "rule," refers to the right of an individual to make informed, voluntary choices for herself, under the influence of as little bias, coercion, pressure or duress as possible. In Western bioethics, a patient's autonomy is typically regarded as the highest priority, and has become the cornerstone of most medical legislation and ethical standards. For example, the UN's Universal Declaration on Bioethics and Human Rights (2005, Article 5) states clearly: "The autonomy of persons to make decisions, while taking responsibility for those decisions and respecting the autonomy of others, is to be respected."

Support for autonomous medical decision-making should occur within the context of the fiduciary relationship, a relationship of implicit two-way trust between the patient and doctor. Our personal autonomy limits the role of others who might influence the patient to make a choice that doesn't reflect their own wishes or best interests.

In clinical practice, blind adherence to public health legislation that runs counter to the patient's choice and/or the doctor's judgment is considered an abrogation of a doctor's duty, even when the legislation is presented as a public good.

The prevailing ethical narrative of the current pandemic is a blend of collectivism and utilitarianism, which states that the right action is the one that will bring about the greatest good for the largest number of people. "We're in this together" and "do your part" are the slogans of this mindset. But as anodyne or benevolent as those slogans sound, we must be wary of the harms that can be allowed, even endorsed, by unreflective public health decision-making with collectivism at its heart, which may appeal to the majority at the expense of the minority.

Nonmaleficence, the Hippocratic Oath in its purest form— "*primum non nocere*" *(first, do no harm)*—is a centrepiece of modern bioethics. Since some persons, such as health-care workers, are in a unique position to be infected and transmit viruses to patients, their families, and the general public (a kind of harm), mandating COVID-19 vaccination for certain sectors of the population would seem at first blush to be justified to reduce dramatically the possibility of harm to others. But the force of protecting the public good becomes less compelling when the principle of nonmaleficence is applied to those individuals, and as data emerges pointing to risk from an unprecedented number of vaccine adverse effects. Furthermore, if we are to be consistent, the *primum non nocere* principle must apply as much to the actions of others that affect me as it does to my actions that affect others; taking a vaccine with possible adverse health effects for myself (so that I might protect others) violates the nonmaleficence principle as much as if my failing to get vaccinated could be shown to cause harm to others. And, as Michael Kowalik elegantly writes,

> It is often overlooked in this normative context that mandatory vaccination violates body autonomy and thus constitutes actual harm (not merely a risk of harm) to any person made to accept vaccination under duress. This type of harm is not negated by any positive health effect of the procedure but constitutes a distinct category; it affects the ontological dimensions of personhood. The threshold of reasonable necessity for medical coercion would have to be proportional to this harm and

supported by a clear causative link between non-vaccination and serious harm to others.[4]

Furthermore, while the implicit 'obligation to vaccinate' fuels much of the pro-vaccine narrative, it is not clear that there is a moral obligation to vaccinate oneself against COVID-19 or that there are sound ethical reasons to mandate vaccination under *any* circumstances, even when a vaccine is medically risk-free. To quote Kowalik again, "mandatory vaccination amounts to discrimination against healthy, innate biological characteristics, which goes against the established norms and is also defeasible a priori."

The fathers of American bioethics, Tom Beauchamp and James Childress, assert that autonomy "is undermined by coercion, persuasion, and manipulation." To make a voluntary choice is, at minimum, to do what you would do in the absence of coercion, persuasion, or manipulation. It is especially important in a medical context that patients make choices based on the perceived intrinsic value of those choices and not for other reasons. It is important that your decision to undergo surgery, for example, is on account of the inherent benefits of the surgery, as you understand them, and not for financial gain or pressure from doctors or the public at large.

Given all of this, it is important to realize that vaccine mandates are, by definition, coercive strategies. They impose a consequence on people who, without the threat of losing their jobs, would not voluntarily choose vaccination. If they would voluntarily agree to vaccination, the mandate would be unnecessary. So keeping your job is now a major consideration in the decision whether to get

4   Kowalik, Michael. "Ethics of Vaccine Refusal" *Journal of Medical Ethics,* 2021, https://jme.bmj.com/content/medethics/early/2021/10/20/medethics-2020-107026.full.pdf. Accessed 19 November 2021.

vaccinated, prompting the ethical question: is it ethically justified to put financial interest at the centre of your medical decision-making, significantly influencing your own autonomous choice?

A common pushback against objections to coercion is the nature of our current circumstances. Pandemics pose a unique ethical challenge, because what one person does potentially affects others, and the impact of one person's actions on others can be grave and substantial. For this reason, there is some historical precedent for mandating vaccines, at least for health-care workers.

Our approach to dealing with smallpox is one of those precedents. It has been suggested that the American case of *Jacobson v. Massachusetts*, from 1905, which saw vaccines successfully mandated to treat a smallpox outbreak, provides good justification for COVID-19 vaccine mandates. In philosophy, we call this an argument from analogy, a type of inductive argument that uses similarities between two cases to infer other shared qualities. For arguments from analogy to work, the analogues must be sufficiently similar. But with *Jacobson* and the COVID-19 pandemic, they clearly are not. The viruses and the vaccines are vastly different in kind. Smallpox is highly virulent with an infection fatality rate more than thirty-times greater than COVID-19.[5] The average age of death from COVID-19 exceeds the national life expectancy, whereas smallpox preyed on the very young (age one to five years)

---

5 This is a very conservative estimate. The numbers, of course, depend on what IFR you use for COVID-19 and there are substantial differences in IFR and infection spread across countries and continents. John Ioannidis estimates a global IFR of 0.15% for COVID-19 across all age groups, which would make smallpox (with an IFR of 30%) 200 times more deadly than COVID-19. (https://pubmed.ncbi.nlm.nih.gov/33768536/) Some seroprevalence data indicate the IFR for COVID-19 is much closer to 0.05%, which would make COVID-19 600 times less deadly than smallpox for healthy individuals under the age of 70. (https://www.ncbi.nlm.nih.gov/pmc/articles/PMC7947934/)

and middle-aged (thirty to sixty years). Furthermore, the smallpox vaccine was a "sterilizing" vaccine, whereas the COVID-19 vaccines are "leaky," meaning that they don't always protect recipients of the vaccine who are exposed to the virus and they permit recipients to be infectious. Furthermore, the virus that causes COVID-19 has been found to infect a wide range of animals, including bats, cats, minks, pangolins and wild deer, whereas smallpox could only spread through human contact. So we can't clearly argue by analogy from the *Jacobson* case that COVID-19 vaccine mandates are justified restrictions on personal autonomy for the sake of public health.

A more recent example of a failed analogy involves the Hepatitis B virus. As with smallpox, the Hepatitis B vaccine also isn't very comparable to the COVID-19 vaccines. As with smallpox, the Hepatitis B vaccine is a sterilizing vaccine that offers robust and lifelong immunity from a chronic infection that is often devastating. Even then, antibodies against the Hepatitis B are typically checked before and after a series of injections to see if further shots are needed. None of these conditions exist with the COVID-19 shots, where serological testing for antibodies against SARS-CoV-2 is largely discouraged.

The mere existence of a vaccine to counter a certain virus does not allow us to assume that the vaccine should therefore be mandated. The following considerations explore some of the nuances of this issue, and are crucial to determining when the threshold has been met to justify ethically mandating COVID-19 vaccination.

Morbidity and mortality: For a vaccine mandate to be ethically justified, the disease in question must be a highly virulent pathogen, which is a significant cause of morbidity and mortality, and it poses a substantial threat to everyone. The mortality rate from smallpox, for example, is approximately 30 per cent. Ebola is also a highly virulent pathogen with an infection fatality rate (IFR) of approximately 50 per cent and is capable of inducing a lethal hemorrhagic fever. COVID-19, by contrast, has an IFR of 0.05 per cent for a healthy person under seventy years of age. Most people who contract the disease experience only minor symptoms. By comparison, at least, to smallpox and Ebola, COVID-19 is not a highly virulent pathogen, and therefore does not obviously meet the epidemiological threshold for morbidity and mortality to justify vaccine mandates.

Availability of effective, approved treatment options: Mandating vaccination would require that no effective and available means exist to treat the disease. This is not the case with COVID-19. Early outpatient treatment options (including but not limited to ivermectin, fluvoxamine, quercetin and even vitamin D3) exist to treat COVID-19.

Whether the vaccine is sterilizing: Since justifying a vaccination mandate depends largely on the effectiveness of the vaccine, and vaccine effectiveness is at least in part a function of its sterilizing capabilities, how sterilizing or non-sterilizing ("leaky") the vaccine is should be crucial to determining the ethical justification of the mandate. Vaccine mandates assume the vaccines prevent transmission of the pathogen. But the mRNA vaccines do not prevent transmission of COVID-19 or infection with the virus. The Director of the CDC, Israel's Director of Public Health, the Chief Scientific Advisor to the UK Government, and even Dr. Fauci are becoming increasingly clear about this. Rather, COVID-vaccinated persons can still become infected with, and transmit, the virus.[6] If we adopt the principle that vaccine effectiveness is at least in part a function of its ability to reduce transmission, then non-sterilizing vaccines are less effective than sterilizing vaccines, and the non-sterilizing COVID-19 vaccines have not clearly met the threshold for efficacy. In fact, as a recent study of 68 countries around the world and 2947 counties within the US shows, higher rates of vaccination do not decrease overall COVID-19 cases. Since the COVID-19 vaccines are not preventing transmission, they must be seen more as personal treatment and less as a public health measure. And if the vaccines are not about public health, then what justifies the mandates? One would think the argument would need to shift to focus instead on the harms of infected people possibly overburdening the health care system, but that is a very different argument, indeed, and not obviously an easy one to make.

A secondary problem is the skewing of the efficacy findings of the vaccines. An editorial in the peer-reviewed journal *Medicine* in February 2021 raised the problem of relative versus absolute risk reduction with respect to the COVID-19 vaccines: "Omitting absolute risk reduction findings in public health and clinical reports of vaccine efficacy . . . ignores unfavorable outcomes and misleads the public's impression and scientific understanding of a treatment's efficacy and benefits."[7] Understanding absolute risk reduction

6 We saw that countries and regions like Israel, UK, Gibraltar, etc. with early vaccination campaigns and high uptake also experienced high COVID-19 case counts and growing deaths. Despite continued insistence that vaccination prevents transmission, Canada is following this pattern, as already evidenced in Toronto's September 15 epidemiological update that shows 45% of deaths over the July 11-Sept 11 period were in fully or partially vaccinated persons. https://gis.blog.ryerson.ca/files/2021/09/Screenshot-2021-09-16-at-11-43-01-COVID-19-Epidemiological-Summary-of-Cases.png. Accessed 22 November 2021.

7 Brown, Ronald. "Outcome Reporting Bias in COVID-19 MRNA Vaccine Clinical Trials," *Medicina,* vol. 57, no. 3, 2021. https://doi.org/10.3390/medicina57030199. Accessed 16 November 2021.

(ARR) versus relative risk reduction (RRR) is not a simple task for the lay person, but the upshot is this. In the case of COVID-19, the difference between ARR and RRR is dramatic. When it is reported that the COVID-19 vaccines have a 94.6% reported efficacy, that sounds like you will reduce your risk of infection and illness by nearly 95% if you get vaccinated. But the high efficacy rate reported in the vaccine studies is a comparison of the ratio of illness prevalence in the treatment and placebo groups (RRR). However, to understand to what degree the vaccines actually reduce the risk of contracting COVID-19, one must examine the ARR value. And according to the Pfizer trial data, their vaccine afforded individuals less than a 1% reduction in the risk of contracting the disease compared to not receiving the vaccine at all. It is for this reason that the FDA clearly states in its *Communicating Risks and* Benefits guidelines: "Absolute risks are always more informative . . . Provide absolute risks, not just relative risks. Patients are unduly influenced when risk information is presented using a relative risk approach; this can result in suboptimal decisions. Thus, an absolute risk format should be used."[8] This information has not, unfortunately, been effectively communicated to Canadians, which further undermines our capacity for informed consent.

The risk/benefit profile: The validity of a vaccination mandate also depends largely on the risks from the disease balanced against the risks from the vaccine used to prevent it. When vaccination benefits are high (because the vaccine effectively prevents infection and

---

8 Fischhoff, B., Brewer, N. T. and Downs, J. S. "Communicating risks and benefits: An evidence-based users' guide. US FDA. 2011. https://www.fda.gov/about-fda/reports/communicating-risks-and-benefits-evidence-based-users-guide. Accessed 23 November 2021.

transmission of a disease with a significant IFR, and there are no known, effective treatments), and the health risks from vaccination are low, mandating vaccination may be justified. That is not the case with COVID-19 vaccines. The virus itself has a comparatively low IFR, the vaccines are non-sterilizing, and there have been an unprecedented number of COVID-19 vaccine harms.[9] The bar we set for benefit over harm simply does not support mandated vaccination.

Disproportionate harms: A vaccination mandate might be ethically justified as long as it does not harm people more than it provides safety or relief from the illness it's supposed to treat. As psychiatrist and psychopharmacologist David Healy said, "A core feature of healthcare is that a medicine should not produce disproportionate problems; a sleeping pill should not cause peripheral neuropathy or birth defects." But the COVID-19 vaccines are showing themselves to produce disproportionate harms. A recently published study in the science journal *Toxicology Reports* showed "very conservatively that there are five times the number of deaths attributable to

9   Kostoff, R., Calina, D., Kanduc, D., Briggs, M., Vlachoyiannopoulos, P., Svistunov, A., Tsatsakis, A. "Why are we vaccinating children against COVID-19?" *Toxicology Reports,* vol. 8, 2021. https://doi.org/10.1016/j.toxrep.2021.08.010. Accessed 29 October 2021. Pfizer's own 6-month trial results show that their COVID vaccine is causing a 300% increase in adverse events, a 75% increase in severe adverse events and a 43% increase in deaths. Classen, J. Bart. "US COVID-19 Vaccines Proven to Cause More Harm than Good Based on Pivotal Clinical Trial Data Analyzed Using the Proper Scientific Endpoint, 'All Cause Severe Morbidity.'" *Trends in Internal Medicine,* vol 1. no. 1, 2021.

As of November 14, 2021, Public Health Ontario reported 537 incidents of myocarditis (inflammation of the heart muscle) or pericarditis (inflammation of the lining around the heart) following receipt of COVID-19 mRNA vaccines in Ontario alone. Depending on the cause and extent of myocardial damage, historically this increases the mortality rate to 20% at 1 year and 50% at 5 years. https://www.publichealthontario.ca/-/media/documents/ncov/epi/covid-19-aefi-report.pdf?sc_lang=en, https://health-infobase.canada.ca/covid-19/vaccine-safety/#detailedSafetySignals

each inoculation vs those attributable to COVID-19 in the most vulnerable 65+ demographic."[10] And, notably, data from the UK Office for National Statistics showed that deaths among teenagers have increased 56 per cent since the COVID-19 vaccine rollout began. Since the risk from COVID-19 itself decreases drastically as age decreases, the longer-term effects of the vaccines on the lower age groups will worsen their risk-benefit ratio, perhaps substantially. Persons in the 25-34 age group, for example, will be more vulnerable to disproportionate harms from vaccine mandates than those in the 65+ group. And, one might argue, they have the most to lose if affected by a vaccine injury since they are at the beginning of their lives and careers, and may have young families to support, or plan to have families in the future. Therefore, COVID-19 vaccination mandates will be potentially more harmful, and therefore less justified, as we work our way down the age groups.

Risk assessment: When it comes to making health care decisions, people vary widely in how they assess risk. Some will opt to take a chance while others will not. Risk averseness depends on many factors, including age and gender, personality, health status, life plans, past experiences, and the existence of family and other relationships. A person with end-stage cancer may be more willing to enroll in a cancer drug trial with unknown or even known severe side effects. A person with a young family may be less likely to take on risks that threaten their employment status. Applying a rule that forces all of us to behave in the same way, assuming the same level of risk, is a further affront to personal autonomy, is ethically unjustified, and is likely to generate much reasonable resistance.

10   Kostoff et al.

* * *

The second aspect of mandating COVID-19 vaccinations that poses a unique ethical challenge has to do with authority and legitimacy. To what extent should the state, as well as private entities, be able to implement measures that protect public health even if the measures violate our personal freedoms?

What makes public health 'public' is that, at least in part, it is the business of public institutions and not just private individuals. Who or what those public institutions are, and what they do to promote the health of populations, is important to understanding how effective or harmful those actions are likely to be. If we assume, in a functional democracy, that action by the government is action by the people, then the interests of the government and the people should align. By extension, the physical and mental well-being of the population should be the sole end of morally responsible public health policy. Policy, again, should align with public interest. In practice, however, the interests of public institutions and legislating bodies may not align with the public interest.

Risks and experimentation: Perhaps the most important ethical consideration of our vaccination mandates relates to the fact that many of the vaccines are novel technologies still in their Phase III clinical trials. And, with the exception of the Cominarty BioNTech COVID-19 vaccine, they are available under emergency use authorization (EUA) only. This means they are investigational by nature, making recipients of COVID-19 vaccines participants in an ongoing research trial.

Ethically, because of the inherent risks of pharmaceutical trial participation, an investigational vaccine should *never* be mandated. Too little is known about the safety and efficacy of the research product, and especially about possible longterm harms, which is why research subjects enjoy enhanced protection. Since unknowns about safety and efficacy enhance risk and undermine autonomous medical decision-making, participants can't give true informed consent in the way they could for tried-and-true pharmaceutical products.

A number of ethical guidelines exist to acknowledge the risks of trial participation and protect participants from them. The most notable of these is the Nuremberg Code, which mandates that medical experimentation on human subjects takes place only in accordance with basic principles that "satisfy moral, ethical, and legal concepts," including proper preparations "to protect the experimental subject against even remote possibilities of injury disability or death." In Canada, the Tri-Council Policy Statement: Ethical Conduct for Research Involving Humans (TCPS 2—2018) was created to promote the ethical conduct of research involving humans.[11] It very specifically and carefully outlines protections for those participating in research involving humans, whether the stated risks are high or where there are substantial unknown risks. History has shown that many of the risks associated with medical research and the long-term harms of some pharmaceuticals are not known until years down the road. In the case of thalidomide, for instance, some of the injuries to the kidneys, heart, reproductive organs, ears and eyes, were not discovered until a decade after release. And Tylenol, a drug that has been on the market for more than half a century and is generally thought to be harmless, was just discovered to increase risk-taking behavior among some users.[12]

11 *Tri-Council Policy Statement: Ethical Conduct for Research Involving Humans — TCPS 2 (2018).* https://ethics.gc.ca/eng/policy-politique_tcps2-eptc2_2018.html. Accessed 22 November, 2021.

12 Keaveney, A., Peters, E., Way, B., "Effects of acetaminophen on risk taking," vol. 15, no. 7, 2020. https://pubmed.ncbi.nlm.nih.gov/32888031/. Accessed 23 November 2021.

Given the lack of public awareness that the COVID-19 vaccines came to market under emergency authorization, and the fact that the COVID-19 vaccination consent forms do not reflect the ethical protections for research participants, it has become clear that genuine fully informed consent is not possible for the COVID-19 vaccines. Can it ever be ethical to mandate that to which a person cannot, in principle, consent?

Integrity of process: In a pandemic situation where the principles of public health must be harnessed quickly in order to secure the best outcome, information transparency is critical. In the ideal situation, there would be no conflicts of interest, and there would be an effective uptake of information at the patient level to assess the vaccines' safety and efficacy. It is important to use and improve available systems like the Vaccine Adverse Event Reporting System (VAERS), and to listen to the reports of ER doctors and nurses, first responders, and family physicians—those on the pandemic's front line—who are most likely to treat the sick. And it is crucial to assume that any adverse medical event, especially in those without pre-existing conditions, could be linked to vaccination until that can be ruled out. But it's not at all clear that is happening. Furthermore, there are serious concerns about the integrity of process in the vaccine trials. As a British Medical Journal November 2021 article states, "A regional director who was employed at the research organisation Ventavia Research Group has told The BMJ that the company falsified data, unblinded patients, employed inadequately trained vaccinators, and was slow to follow up on adverse events reported in Pfizer's pivotal phase III trial."[13] The capacity for an individual to consent to taking

---

13   Thacker, P. "Covid-19: Researcher Blows the Whistle on Data Integrity Issues in Pfizer's Vaccine Trial." *Social Cognitive and Affective Disorder,* vol. 15, no. 7, 2020, https://pubmed.ncbi.nlm.nih.gov/32888031/. Accessed 20 November, 2021.

one of the COVID-19 vaccines depends substantially on the integrity of the trial process; without this, it is unclear how any person who takes one of the COVID-19 vaccines could give full and informed consent. The difficulty of establishing a clear causative link between the COVID-19 vaccines and late-onset health conditions, and the fact that the vaccine manufacturers are typically not liable for the adverse effects of their products, allows the industry to prioritize profits over consumer safety. This is a moral hazard that we should be very careful to avoid.

Regulatory capture: To borrow an example from across the border, the American managed care giant Kaiser Permanente is one of the largest employers enacting a vaccination mandate for its 300,000 employees. While Kaiser claims that it is simply following Center for Disease Control (CDC) guidelines in mandating vaccinations, Kaiser actually has an integral role in creating those guidelines. It is the predominant member of the CDC's Vaccine Safety Datalink (VSD) collaborative project, and a leading member on the Advisory Committee on Immunization Practices (ACIP). This leaves the company in a significant decision-making position (it had already recommended to the CDC that the vaccines be granted emergency authorization). Kaiser's role demonstrates that the two chief public health institutions in the United States, the CDC and FDA, are not impartial independent decision-makers guiding public health policies. They are heavily influenced by entities with financial interests that potentially conflict with the public good, and they are overseeing a top-down flow of information with very little uptake of information from frontline workers and vaccine recipients. Another example of this kind of regulatory capture is evident in a video recently released by Health Canada, which encourages COVID-19 vaccination. It was produced by "19 to Zero," which describes itself as an independent, non-profit organization but its sponsors include the Vaccine Confidence Project, Pfizer, Moderna, and GSK.

Conflicts of interest versus bias: It is important to note that the presence of competing interests does not necessarily create bias in decision-making. A corporation can have a financial interest in a certain outcome without being motivated primarily by that interest. And a corporation can benefit financially from an outcome without doing so primarily because of its financial interest. Take, for example, the case of Merck Pharmaceuticals and penicillin. In 1942, after Anne Miller became the first American to be successfully treated with the new antibiotic, Merck shared the secrets of how to make penicillin with its competitors so the drug could be produced on a large scale. The move helped save many lives during WWII. Problems arise, however, when regulatory bodies are financially incentivized to do what is not clearly in the interest of public health. This "regulatory capture" can ultimately harm persons and can make mandates appear more scientifically, legally, and ethically justified than they are.

The example of opioids: There are very clear historical examples of medical regulatory capture in which FDA, CDC, and Data and Safety Monitoring oversight have been overly influenced by the pharmaceutical industry. The recent opioid epidemic, fueled by the overprescribing of oxycodone, fentanyl, and other painkillers, is a prime example. Although the abundance of harm is clear—according to the CDC, more than 500,000 American lives have been lost from overdoses involving opioids since 1999, and the lives of many more have been devastated—that harm has been obscured by the efforts of the pharmaceutical industry that helped to shape patient perceptions of pain, risk, and addiction, and influence how doctors think about the safety and effectiveness of these drugs.

Purdue, the company that makes OxyContin, aggressively promoted its use, courting doctors with promotional material and gifts to make ever-more use of the drug despite its demonstrated harm and a lack of increased efficacy.[14] Court documents showed that Purdue spent $207 million US on advertising and sponsored 20,000 pain "education programs," engaging key opinion leaders to defend OxyContin's safety and efficacy. Five years after its release, OxyContin generated an annual revenue of more than $1 billion.

Unfortunately, it seems that the FDA may not have learned a lesson from the opioid epidemic. According to a 2020 article in the American Medical Association's *Journal of Ethics*, "Despite this mounting criticism, FDA policies for approving and labeling opioids remain largely unchanged. The FDA has not undertaken a root cause analysis of its regulatory errors that contributed to this public health catastrophe, let alone instituted any major reforms. To the contrary, the agency has adopted a defensive posture and sought to shift blame."

The case of SSRIs: Another example of pharmaceutical regulatory capture is the over-prescribing of selective serotonin reuptake inhibitors (SSRIs), especially for adolescents. A study published in the *British Medical Journal*, which examined documents from seventy different double-blind, placebo-controlled trials of SSRIs, and serotonin and norepinephrine reuptake inhibitors

---

14 Van Zee, A. "The Promotion and Marketing of OxyContin: Commercial Triumph, Public Health Tragedy." *American Journal of Public Health,* vol. 99, no. 2, 2009, https://www.ncbi.nlm.nih.gov/pmc/articles/PMC2622774/. Accessed 19 November 2021.

(SNRIs), showed that pharmaceutical companies underreported information regarding the full extent of serious harm in clinical study reports. These reports were sent to major health authorities like the FDA. An independent review found that the commonly prescribed SSRI Paxil is not safe for teenagers, even though a 2001 GlaxoSmithKline-funded drug trial employed these same findings to market Paxil as perfectly safe for teenagers. This sort of thing is hardly anomalous. Dr. Richard Horton, the current editor-in-chief of *The Lancet*, writes: "The case against science is straightforward: much of the scientific literature, perhaps half, may simply be untrue. Afflicted by studies with small sample sizes, tiny effects, invalid exploratory analyses, and flagrant conflicts of interest, together with an obsession for pursuing fashionable trends of dubious importance, science has taken a turn towards darkness." Horton's counterpart at the *New England Journal of Medicine* drew the same conclusion.

The important lesson from the opioid epidemic and SSRI prescription cases is that the regulatory climate in the US heading into 2020 was primed for another instance of regulatory capture of exactly the sort we are seeing with the COVID vaccines.

Historical examples, such as the over-prescribing of opioids and SSRIs, serve as reminders of what can happen when government institutions are overly influenced by the pharmaceutical industry, and of the downstream harms that can happen when human health decisions are subject to the profit motive.

According to Harvard professor of medicine and former editor-in-chief of the *New England Journal of Medicine*, Arnold Seymour Relman, "The medical profession is being bought by the pharmaceutical industry, not only in terms of the practice of medicine but also in terms of teaching and research." The regulatory climate in the US was certainly primed for another instance of regulatory capture of exactly the sort we are seeing with the COVID-19 vaccination mandates. And it is not clear that corporate entities, our public health officials or the media have provided sufficient evidence to show that the non-sterilizing COVID-19 vaccines reach the threshold of ethical justification in order for them to be mandated.

* * *

One step removed from the active influence we are seeing with Big Pharma is the more subtle, perhaps insidious, efforts of the state to influence public behaviour under the banner of the common good.

Governments in several western countries, including Canada, have formed what are colloquially referred to as "nudge" units, teams of people schooled in behavioural science who both monitor public sentiment and plan ways to shape it in accord with government policy.

The concept was born out of *Nudge*, a 2008 book by Richard Thaler and Cass Sunstein, which posited using behavioural science to both understand how people think and to influence them to make better choices. Better for themselves and, ostensibly, for society as a whole.

"People often make poor choices—and look back at them with bafflement!" Thaler and Sunstein write. "We do this because as human beings, we all are susceptible to a wide array of routine biases that can lead to an equally wide array of embarrassing blunders in education, personal finance, health care, mortgages and credit cards, happiness, and even the planet itself."

Sunstein now heads up a World Health Organization advisory group focusing on behaviour related to COVID-19. And officials within Canada's own nudge unit acknowledge our federal government is a global leader in embracing the WHO approach to understanding and influencing pandemic sentiment and actions.

Dr. Theresa Tam, Canada's chief public health officer, praised Canada's use of the nudge approach as a way to address the problem of "vaccine hesitancy." It was notable for being one of the rare occasions public officials have acknowledged the behaviour-studying unit inside government.

"Some of the studies are actually carried out by the Privy Council Office, where there is a behavioural insight team," Tam said, as reported by the *Toronto Star*. "We do know that the intention for Canadians to get the vaccine is actually quite high and I think has improved since we started the vaccine campaign itself."

The FDA's risk communication document (mentioned earlier in this chapter) states very clearly: "we recommend ways to *nudge* individuals towards better comprehension and greater welfare."[15]

Defenders of the nudge approach will say it's permissible to manipulate, even coerce, behaviour if its goal is making people do the right thing, act in accordance with truth, save them from themselves. But that poses an intriguing question: are we entitled to make our own choices only as long as they are the 'right' ones? Who determines what's 'right'? And what tests do we apply do determine it? Truth? Popular opinion? What the group perceives to be best for itself? What the leader of the group demands?

Even if individuals do make mistakes, or choose what is collectively deemed wrong, is that a good enough reason to nudge their decisions? What do autonomy and freedom of choice look like if we are only ever able to select from a narrow set of options and then nudged towards one over the others? Are we really free in that

---

15 https://www.fda.gov/about-fda/reports/communicating-risks-and-benefits-evidence-based-users-guide. Accessed 20 November 2021.

condition? What will our democracy look like if we are not creating government but rather following the nudges of government?

The nudge approach also assumes that experts know best. The aforementioned Dr. Tam is one of them. But what does it mean to be an expert in the context of the pandemic? And how should engaged, informed, and free people view experts and their advice?

The irrepressible Nobel laureate Richard Feynman had a healthy skepticism of experts. In a speech to the National Science Teachers Association, he said science teaches us not to embrace the experts, but to doubt them. "Science is the belief in the ignorance of experts. When someone says 'science teaches such-and-such,' he is using the word incorrectly. Science doesn't teach it; experience teaches it." It follows that skepticism of experts is evidence of a truly scientific mind.

The concept of expert has changed over time, resulting in today's version of hyper-specialized authority. There are no more polymaths. While experts may have deep knowledge and insight in their own fields, their narrow perspectives can be poison for public policy. Someone steeped in the intricacies of human immunology may be able to evaluate spike protein production but will have little insight into the effects of a comprehensive lockdown on the economy. Even if confined to the realm of public health, epidemiological experts who have recommended all kinds of policies that limit public interaction and isolate whole populations have little to say about the psychological fallout of those policies. We hear far more today about daily positive COVID-19 test results than we do about youth suicide rates, the likely fallout of isolating mandates.

Beyond doubting the ability of experts, critics of the nudge approach often rely on the idea that nudges violate autonomy and that "nobody knows better than I do what's best for me." But that isn't my defence. First, that is probably false: we pretty clearly make decisions that are not, even by our own measure, best for ourselves. I don't think we ought to respect autonomy because the individual is necessarily the best personal authority. We ought to respect autonomy for two other reasons. One, it is the individual, alone, who will have to bear the consequences of her (in this case, medical) choices. And two, there is value in having the space to shape, and be the author of, one's own life even if someone else could have written the chapters of that life better.

There is, to put it very simply, value in having a nation of free people.

CHAPTER 5

A WAY FORWARD

I have filled many previous pages with an overview of the problems created by our response to COVID-19 and the challenges the response has posed to me and to our society as a whole. Is it enough to simply detail our shortcomings, our errors, even the potential malice that lies beneath policy and popular reaction?

No. Part of the journey I've been on these past months has also been one of discovery, of seeing potential solutions and pathways that would allow us to move forward together. In these final chapters of my book, I'd like to detail them. The first suite of prescriptions is focused on the bigger picture, on whole populations rather than individuals (although individual action is required to affect the bigger picture). The second, in the next chapter, deals with advice for you, the reader. What can you do, now, to make a difference in your own life, the lives of those in your immediate circle? And then how does that make an impact on the larger world?

First, I think we need to remember, as cliché as it might sound, that our circumstances don't need to define us, however regrettable, unfathomable, or unrelenting those circumstances may be. We need to embrace the authorship of our own lives and our communities and design our steps forward. We can be shaped and refined without being defined by our circumstances.

I remember reading with great sadness that aboriginal people who have suffered at the hands of colonization live with a sense of "perpetual grief" owing to the still-unresolved dispossession of their lands, suppression of culture, and other affronts to their history, identity, and well-being. Their grief is so enduring, framing each of their steps forward, that it seems to have come to define them and often overtakes them. And I remember wondering if this is inevitable.

Then I happened upon this year's recipient of the Nobel Prize for Literature and was struck by how he wrote about his experiences. Abdulrazak Gurnah fled Zanzibar in the 1960s after the revolution and moved to Canterbury, UK. In Zanzibar, "Terror ruled our lives" he wrote. But "[r]acism was pervasive when I came to Britain. You couldn't get a bus without encountering something that made you recoil." He writes that the Britain he arrived in was so white that, when he caught a glimpse of himself in a shop window, he wondered for a moment who he was. Before arriving in the UK, Gurnah had formed an image of the country as one of "courtesy and politeness." He had no hint of the hostility he would meet. He encountered "bad words, ugly stares, rudeness," and endured poverty and homesickness in a foreign land. But he says the characters in his stories are "shaped but not defined" by circumstances, much like himself. David Pilling says of *Afterlives,* Gurnah's latest novel, "a girl is beaten up by her adopted parents because she has secretly learnt how to read. Yet she goes on to woo the young man who will become her husband, to crack jokes and to live a life defined by her own will."

Each set of stories has its own complexities and I have surely glossed over these here, but it seems to me, in very broad strokes, that one is a tale of success in terms of recovery from deep societal trauma, while the other is not.

The harms caused by the pandemic response, in important ways, are likely different from the harms in these stories. But perhaps we can still learn something from them. If the pandemic response does involve democratic, scientific, journalistic missteps, how can we correct these? How can we get ourselves on a better track? How can we recalibrate and best emerge from the ashes?

Let's start with the bigger picture. I wish to boil down the next few thousand words into a manageable prescription, namely this: we all need to become thoroughgoing skeptics in the truest classical sense of the word. We need to lose our fear of asking questions, of noting when statements are inconsistent or don't agree with common sense. And we especially have to withdraw the automatic trust that is all too eagerly awarded to people and institutions that have yet to earn the trust. Or, worse, had our trust but lost it.

We need to become committed skeptics when it comes to some key concepts, and towards important constructs and institutions that affect our lives daily. First, the concepts:

We must become more skeptical of our concepts of experts and expertise: look critically at who they are and what the term means, and what scope of action we grant the experts.

We must become more skeptical of academia: realize that far too many campuses have become monocultures promoting a particular set of values and beliefs, and more interested in stifling dissent than cultivating and examining it.

We must become more skeptical of media: understand there has been a fundamental shift in newsrooms away from the traditional standards of objectivity and balance, toward the promotion of narratives and the stifling of dissent, akin to what we see on today's campuses.

We must become more skeptical of government: understand the pandemic has elevated government figures into positions that are all too often beyond reproach, and policies stemming from these figures are sheathed in the armour of 'collective good' which shields them from honest analysis and criticism.

Above all, we must become more skeptical of consensus, or the wisdom of the masses. On Emirates flight 203 in September 2018, some passengers began showing flu-like symptoms. When other passengers observed these symptoms, they started to feel sick as well, and such a panic broke out that the whole flight was quarantined upon arrival in New York City. The investigation afterwards revealed that only a few passengers were actually sick. Indeed, diseases and the atmosphere of disease is a fertile ground for mass hysteria to develop. Humans are fallible, even more when we act as a group. To quote Agent K from the sci-fi classic *Men in Black*, "A *person* is smart. *People* are dumb, panicky, dangerous animals and you know it."

Now let's look at each of those prescriptions individually, starting with experts and expertise. The word *expert* comes from the Latin *expertus*, meaning "tried, proved, known by experience." The roots are interesting: *peritus* means "experienced, tested," a suffixed form of the root *per-* "to try, risk." There is a connection to the idea that an expert is someone who is, or has, tested or been tested, and also is willing to try or risk. There is, therefore, a sense of creativity or imagination, or at least openness, in the notion of being an expert. Also interesting is the fifteenth-century sense of *expert* as a "person wise through experience."

Is this how we conceive of experts now? I don't think so. Experts today are seen as people with extremely specialized knowledge that makes them authorities on matters pertaining to their specialty. We have even coined the term "subject matter experts" (SMEs) to refer to those highly sought after persons with specialized knowledge of a particular field. But where is the wisdom? Where is the experience?

Where is the sense of having been tested? Of being willing to test one's knowledge, to try, to risk. These are characteristics indicative of an openness, a sense of humility, and possibly more: being a brave and creative thinker.

Worse, we treat words like *science* and *expert* as synonyms for perfection. And we idolize those concepts. I'm not sure we know what they mean, but we idolize them nonetheless. And we've taken it further and grafted new moral meaning onto those concepts.

If you're on the so-called side of science and the experts, you are not only on the right side intellectually, but you are virtuous, you are morally good, you are a fine citizen, and an upstanding democratic participant. If you are not on the side of the scientists and the experts (and who decides that?), not only are you wrong but you're shut down, excluded, and your voice no longer matters. You are ostracized as surely as the true subjects in the Asch experiment felt they were ostracized (more on this below).

When you listen to the public messaging around the nature of science today, you'd be forgiven for thinking that science is a perfect, closed system devoid of experimentation. There is much talk of "settled science" not just concerning the pandemic but in areas such as climate change or gender.

But science is almost never settled. It is, instead, a process of continual refinement through experimentation, and each experiment holds (at least should hold) the possibility of destroying the entire framework. The element of risk is always there. It also entails exposure, the potential to realize that the theory you've spent the past three months or three years perfecting was actually wrong. Not every attempt to validate a hypothesis will be successful, and some may reveal that a massive rethink is in order. And that's exactly how it should be.

As an ethicist, I'm very concerned about informed consent. When we close off the possibility of informed consent (sometimes before we know everything) and give people the impression that the science is settled—telling them, for example, that there are no safe and effective treatments for COVID-19, or that the vaccines are perfectly safe and effective—we undermine people's ability to weigh options and conduct their own risk/benefit analyses. That is the foundation of informed consent, a deeply entrenched Canadian right. The transparency, or lack thereof, of science and medicine deeply affects our ability to make choices about our own bodies. Further down the line, it affects what kind of lives we will be able to lead and ultimately what democracy looks like.

The other disturbing aspect of recent concepts surrounding expertise is that expertise in one field seems to suffice as expertise in general. But there are problems with assuming that expertise is transferrable in this way.

Doctors like Theresa Tam and Anthony Fauci may be accomplished medical professionals who have specialized knowledge of virology and immunology. But they are not experts in public policy. Their expertise in judging the effects of vaccine mandates or social lockdowns does not extend much further than their labs or offices. As far as we know, they have little expertise in the economic fallout from lockdowns, the social disconnect caused by denying physical contact between a daughter and her elderly father dying in a nursing home, the impact on a six-year-old's education and social development when school is reduced to a never-ending series of Zoom calls. Yet their influence extends to the highest levels of power, and they've attained an odd level of hero worship, if social media is any kind of popular bellwether.

To have the kind of expertise that can take all relevant factors into account, you'd have to be a polymath, someone along the lines of an Aristotle, a Leonardo, a Ben Franklin. I don't know if any of those exist today.

That's dangerous because what's dominating our narrative now is this idea that only experts are allowed to make decisions, but what allows you to become an expert is that you become so narrowly focused on something that it's tough to understand if you could really contextualize what you know in relation to other important spheres of life.

We now have an inability to reconcile or integrate information that's different in kind. For instance, when it became clear recently that there's a mental health crisis among Britain's youth, it didn't get the media uptake that it should have. It certainly didn't become part of the public health discussion. It wasn't integrated into the awareness of the cost of our anti-COVID measures. I think that's largely because the information is different in kind from the standard COVID-related data: new cases, hospitalizations, intensive-care occupancy rates, deaths, and vaccination rates. We've just lost that ability to be able to synthesize disparate genres of information.

We need to get it back. Or, at the least, we need to recognize this shortcoming and build strategies to overcome it.

* * *

When I was a graduate student many years ago, a number of us were focused on ancient Greek philosophy. My supervisor at the time formed what we affectionately called the "Greek gang" and we would gather regularly at his house for dinner and discussion. After dinner, someone would read a paper and we would talk symposium-style for several hours into the evening.

It was wonderful and enriching and inspiring. We all said at the time that we got a lot from those evenings—we learned so much more from them than we did any of our classes. We all thought we were living the ideal of the academy. But it turned out to be an anomaly, a false view of what the academic world is really like, especially today.

When my supervisor retired, the university hired a cohort of new, younger professors to take the place of those like him. Lots of publications and citations under their names, very centred on themselves and their progress towards amassing the litany of accomplishments necessary for promotion and tenure these days. Most want no part of the collegial, extracurricular experience we'd all been enjoying. There was a palpable shift away from a culture where ideas were meant to be shared, examined, debated, and, if necessary, modified or discarded altogether.

It turns out our little circle was not alone. Universities today have become monocultures, dominated by various strands of left-leaning thought that include several variations of critical theory. Certain received wisdoms are now beyond challenge: safety culture dominates and the prevailing idea is that disagreements or unorthodox thought is somehow dangerous, rather than debatable; due process is all too often seen as a sign of privilege and dominance rather than fairness; mob-based bullying is accepted and used as a tool to flush unorthodox ideas and the people who harbour them from campus.

These aren't theoretical musings. The exile of noted academics like Bret Weinstein and Heather Heying from Evergreen College in Washington, or the confrontation between students and Yale professor Nicholas Christakis over the issue of appropriate Halloween costumes, demonstrate the dangerous power and homogenizing effects student-led mobs can wield.

My own experience at Huron College reinforces the notion that the academy is not a place for lively discussion and exploration of ideas. I received no support from colleagues and, worse, no offers to discuss my position, unless you can characterize the largely *ad hominem* Twitter critiques as an attempt at academic discourse.

Can this devolution in academic culture be fixed? I have my doubts, certainly in the near term. So, if the problems with institutions of higher learning today are intractable and if they are deeply connected to the problems at the root of the pandemic response, then perhaps envisioning new arenas for learning is an important way forward.

Decentralizing the process of learning is something we need to explore, including detaching the places of learning from institutions that are primarily structured as corporations framed primarily by their financial interests. I am not alone in pushing this idea.

Former *New York Times* journalist Bari Weiss, herself an exile from the mainstream corporate news industry, has proposed a new university in Austin, Texas focused on the ideals of the Enlightenment, including diversity of thought and academic freedom. The new University of Austin already has a board of more than thirty prominent academics and public figures, including Harvard president emeritus Larry Summers and Pulitzer-winning playwright David Mamet. More than 3,000 professors and PhD holders have inquired about joining its faculty.

Other initiatives include an online university spearheaded by New York University professor Mark Crispin Miller (who many consider a fringe academic because of his vaccine skepticism and promotion of several conspiracy theories), as well as The Democracy Fund's own Ideas Institute initiative here in Canada.

* * *

"How to talk about vaccines with anti-vaxxers, deniers, and belligerent uncles at Thanksgiving" is the headline for a recent story on the website of the Poynter Institute, widely regarded in the news industry as the premiere training ground for journalists. That is a headline designed to treat the other side, vaccine or vaccine-mandate skeptics, with a heavy dose of contempt followed by a booster shot of alienation. There's no assumption that the other side could have even a single point of legitimate doubt. Even though the story itself is far less us-vs-them than the headline, Poynter evidently found the headline appropriate, even laudable.

This is the kind of sentiment being pushed by corporate media, the same media that has seen its trust levels plummet throughout the west in the past decade. The infusion of narrative over honesty, the removal of objectivity from newsrooms, the infusion of bias in every part of the newsgathering process has contributed to the drop in public trust.

A recent investigation by the online news organization *The Markup* is revealing in its inherent bias towards big institutions, the sort of organizations journalists used to target in their role as watchdogs.

The Markup bills itself as "a non-profit newsroom that investigates how powerful institutions are using technology to change our society."

The investigation took to task a report generated by Facebook that defended the social media giant's content profile. According to *The Markup*, Facebook said "the most popular informational content . . . came from sources like UNICEF, ABC News, or the CDC." But an investigation revealed instead that "outlets like *The Daily Wire*, *The Western Journal*, and *BuzzFeed*'s viral content arm were among the top-viewed domains . . ."

Let's break that down. *The Markup* is essentially saying giant organizations like the United Nations, the US government, and ABC News are *a priori* trustworthy while outlets that openly declare a political bias yet do original reporting like *The Daily Wire* are not.

This is a stunning turnaround of priorities for a newsroom. Journalists now defend big government and corporate media (or at least give them a pass) rather than viewing their statements and practices skeptically. How on earth did that evolution (really a de-evolution) occur?

Much of it began with academia. Less than two years ago, University of British Columbia professors Candis Callison and Mary Lynn Young wrote *Reckoning: Journalism's Limits and Possibilities*, which advocated abandoning the ideal of objectivity in journalism. Objectivity, it is argued, is an illusion and, when pursued, is simply a tool to uphold a systemically racist culture dominated by white men. This sentiment, alive in newsrooms long before Callison and Young's book was published, continues to percolate. Objectivity is a dying principle within our traditional media world.

But the traditional media world itself is dying, a victim of its own hubris, its financial arrogance, and a stunning inability to self-reflect. Which is why some journalists with impressive pedigrees are starting to push back. Some who used to ply their trade with old media have left their dying outlets and moved to the greener pastures of independence.

The aforementioned Bari Weiss is one of them. She has now found a lucrative home on the online platform Substack. She has been followed by journalists like Matt Taibbi, former rising star at *Rolling Stone*, Glenn Greenwald, co-founder of *The Intercept* (who left the publication in 2020), and Andrew Sullivan, a former stalwart at *The Atlantic*. All are decidedly heterodox in their outlook, all are practicing fresh and insightful journalism, and I think all are the vanguard of a new direction for the news industry.

* * *

As someone born in the 1970s, there have been moments when government actions have really terrified me but I have never seen popular opinion align with them, even push for them, as strongly as we're seeing now. I think, charitably, what someone might say to that is, "well hold on a minute here, rights are all well and good when things are functioning well, and when we have the luxury to have them. But we're in a crisis here. And we need to think about the greater good. And so, we all need to make sacrifices and we need to put limitations on those rights in order to prevent something terrible from happening, like all of us get sick and die."

As a student of the history of philosophy, I look to British philosopher Thomas Hobbes, who explains that humans form societies because we desire to get out of the state of nature, where we feel vulnerable. In his landmark 1651 treatise on politics, *Leviathan*, he describes life without social structure this way: "No arts; no letters; no society; and which is worst of all, continual fear, and danger of violent death: and the life of man, solitary, poor, nasty, brutish and short." So, humans thought, let's put some limitations on our freedoms in order to protect ourselves a bit more.

But now we're finding ourselves victimized by the very people we expect to support us, and the rights that are supposed to protect us have been turned against us. We are left with a kind of limp, illiberal democracy.

When it comes to public health concerns that by definition involve government, we need to be able to see that state actions may not always be in our best interest, no matter what government officials or their supporters in media say. We need to take a cue from the research ethics concept of "clinical equipoise."

A little etymology is again in order: *equipoise* has meant a sense of *steadiness, balance, equilibrium, composure* since the seventeenth century. It springs from the idea that there is genuine uncertainty within the expert medical community over whether a treatment will be beneficial, and this uncertainty allows for a kind of humility needed to be "on the lookout" for emergent harms from the treatment in question.

Although the term is most commonly used in contemporary ethics, its active use dates back to the late eighteenth century and its context is the granddaddy of all pandemic fears: smallpox. In 1798, Dr. Edward Jenner published his famous defense of vaccinating against smallpox, a truly deadly disease that posed an existential threat to entire populations. Jenner reasoned vaccination offered better protection against the disease than the only alternative preventative measure at the time. "Such work requires the doctor to be in doubt as to which treatment is better," Jenner wrote, "to be in 'equipoise.'" It appears to be the first time the word was used in a medical context. Interestingly, Jenner said he was not himself in a state of equipoise since it was clear to him that vaccinating against smallpox was the best choice (which it probably was). Nevertheless, the first medical mention of this concept comes from what is perhaps our most well-known historical example of mandated vaccination.

It seems to me that we lack this kind of uncertainty when discussing whether COVID-19 vaccines are safe and effective. We instead have a hubris that prevails even in light of recent statements by public health leadership (Dr. Fauci, the director of the CDC, the UK's chief scientific advisor) that the vaccines don't significantly reduce transmission and aren't working quite as well as expected. There is no sense of equipoise when considering whether existing pharmaceuticals and nutraceuticals can effectively treat the infection;

rather, there is certainty paired with ridicule of those who advocate alternatives.

Therefore, it isn't surprising that we lack the humility and the position of equipoise necessary for an awareness of the harms that our current pandemic response may be doing.

The lack of humility has an even darker companion: a censorious streak that seeks to silence voices of dissent. Although I can still get my message out on some social platforms and via special interest groups, posting COVID-19 heresies on places like Twitter, YouTube, and Facebook will often trigger automatic warning tags, de-monetization penalties, and a concerted digital effort to limit visibility and the ability to view and share.

Again, this is done under the aegis of safety. But the health of a society depends as much on freedom of thought as it does on vaccinating otherwise healthy fifteen-year-olds.

John Stuart Mill was perhaps the staunchest advocate for free expression of any western philosopher. The heir apparent to Jeremy Bentham and the concept of utilitarianism, Mill recognized the harm done when free expression is suppressed:

> The peculiar evil of silencing the expression of an opinion is, that it is robbing the human race; posterity as well as the existing generation; those who dissent from the opinion, still more than those who hold it. If the opinion is right, they are deprived of the opportunity of exchanging error for truth: if wrong, they lose, what is almost as great a benefit, the clearer perception and livelier impression of truth, produced by its collision with error.

Note that Mill is just as focused on the rights of citizens to hear questionable speech as he is on the rights of citizens to utter it.

Denying me the right to hear or read is at least as damaging as muzzling me, because it puts constraints on my knowledge.

He also recognized the value of dissent and maintained that it is the eccentrics in society who keep the pulse of civic discourse alive. Today, it is the eccentrics who are labelled dangerous and face attacks against their intelligence and their character, rather than the substance of their arguments. Turning again to Mill:

> In this age, the mere example of non-conformity, the mere refusal to bend the knee to custom, is itself a service. Precisely because the tyranny of opinion is such as to make eccentricity a reproach, it is desirable, in order to break through that tyranny, that people should be eccentric. Eccentricity has always abounded when and where strength of character has abounded; and the amount of eccentricity in a society has generally been proportional to the amount of genius, mental vigor, and moral courage which it contained. That so few now dare to be eccentric marks the chief danger of the time.

I have been thinking about why the responses to criticizing the government and its attendant "experts" have been so strong. Why should disagreement elicit such disdain, shaming, and dismissal rather than just something more benign like, "well, that's an interesting point but I think it doesn't take into account x, y, or z"? Why have we lost our civility when it comes even to asking these kinds of questions?

I have a couple of possible answers.

The first is heresy. Galileo and Copernicus were vilified for their theories because they challenged the prevailing orthodoxy, which was based on the teachings of the Catholic Church. So, it made sense for them to be accused of heresy. But it seems the nature of today's response has a similar feel. Is this because science is the new divine order of experts and to challenge it is as disrespectful as being a heretic? Are our public health officials the 'priests' of this new divine order? If so, to challenge the experts is not just to be guilty of some kind of epistemological hubris but to question those who are supposed to mediate or translate the divine truths about the world for the rest of us. Questioning Drs. Tam and Moore is just as blasphemous as Copernicus challenging the magister of the holy palace in the sixteenth century. And the costs now are just as great as they were then. And think of the consequences and the loss for those who lose belief in their religion. The period after that sort of "belief adjustment," that kind of paradigm shift in one's overarching system of belief, is a terrifying free-fall. That level of discomfort may even make doubting not worth doing in the first place.

The second is terrorism. Is the concern that challenging the prevailing narrative will undermine, and ultimately threaten, people's safety? That it will terrorize them psychologically in addition to posing a physical threat? *Terrorism* is a massively charged word, but I wonder if that is the implicit concern: that challenging the narrative, challenging authority, will harm people. If so, the dissenters are not just guilty of an epistemological failure (to see the truth) but a moral wrong bordering on evil. If the prevailing belief is that the narrative is infallible, that its defenders are pure and altruistic, and that the population's health and survival is at stake, then the dissenters and questioners would seem to be no different than terrorists trying to wreak havoc on civil society.

I don't have a conclusive answer. But it's clear that when we question the narrative, and therefore its defenders, we are doing much more than just questioning. We seem to be threatening the very foundations of who we are as a people. And in the eyes of the defenders, that can't be tolerated.

* * *

I'm about to introduce an idea that uses an allusion to Nazi Germany to make its point. I do so not as an act of hyperbole to grab your attention (you're already deep into this book!) but to demonstrate a crucial parallel: many in our current culture are approaching the existence of unjust rules and practices in the same fashion the broad bureaucracy of totalitarian states in the not-too-distant past approached their unjust, even criminal, rules and practices.

I fully realize the peril in invoking what's known in the online community as Godwin's Law (the longer an argument runs on, the greater the chance someone or something will be compared to Hitler). I've already been attacked on Twitter for using the analogy in an earlier speech: "Time the spoiled adult children grew up and learned about societal responsibility. Drawing any parallels to the Nazi regime is infantile, ridiculous, and low. #COVIDIOTS"

But bear with me as I explain. Almost sixty years ago, Hannah Arendt wrote one of the seminal analyses of the kind of people who made up the machinery of the Final Solution. *Eichmann in Jerusalem: A Report on the Banality of Evil* was spawned from her coverage of the trial of Adolf Eichmann, one of the most wanted Nazis who escaped Europe after Germany's surrender in 1945 and was living a quiet anonymous life in Argentina. Captured by Israeli agents in 1960, he was taken back to Jerusalem, where he faced a very public trial. Eichmann was found guilty of war crimes and hanged two years later.

Arendt covered his trial and was fascinated by the fact Eichmann seemed nothing like the kind of larger-than-life villain one often expects to be at the epicentre of historic evil. After all, the uber-villain is a staple of our history (Genghis Khan, Ivan the

Terrible, Hitler) and our culture (Satan, Moriarty, Darth Vader). Eichmann was unlike any of them. An unassuming technocrat who invoked the classic "just following orders," he exemplified more than anything that evil could be the product of simply not thinking about one's actions. Wrote Arendt:

> For when I speak of the banality of evil, I do so only on the strictly factual level, pointing to a phenomenon which stared one in the face at the trial. Eichmann was not Iago and not Macbeth, and nothing would have been farther from his mind than to determine with Richard III 'to prove a villain.' Except for an extraordinary diligence in looking out for his personal advancement, he had no motives at all . . . He merely, to put the matter colloquially, never realized what he was doing . . . It was sheer thoughtlessness—something by no means identical with stupidity—that predisposed him to become one of the greatest criminals of that period.

Arendt contended that Eichmann wasn't alone in his pedestrian profile. She knew that many in the Nazi apparatus (perhaps most) weren't innate sadists, but were "terribly and terrifyingly normal. From the viewpoint of our legal institutions and of our moral standards of judgment, this normality was much more terrifying than all the atrocities put together."

We needn't focus on the Nazis, or on the atrocities committed during the Holocaust, as our sole analog for the role that the bureaucratic mindset and diffusion of responsibility play in opening the door to harmful acts in the name of public good. Anna Funder's book *Stasiland: Stories from Behind the Berlin Wall* details the culture of control and secrecy in Cold War-era East Germany and deals with precisely the same set of circumstances:

I wonder how it worked inside the Stasi (East German secret police): who thought up these blackmail schemes? Did they send them up the line for approval? Did pieces of paper come back initialled and stamped 'Approved': the ruining of a marriage, the destruction of a career, the imprisonment of a wife, the abandonment of a child? Did they circulate internal updates: 'Five new and different ways to break a heart'?"

The period immediately following the Second World War was alive with psychological studies aimed at explaining the appalling human behaviour from which the world had just emerged. A lot needed to be explained, most of all, how an apex civilization like Germany (the world's first social democracy at the forefront of science, art, culture, and technology) could become the archetype of evil in less than two generations.

Two psychology experiments conducted in the post-war United States were revelatory, and many still believe their conclusions are universally applicable and relevant today. I'll summarize each.

The Asch experiments. Just six years after the end of the Second World War, psychologist Solomon Asch contributed a classic study of group influence on individuals. Asch was interested in how and to what extent people react to group pressure. In the introduction to his work, Asch reviewed the enormously important issue of propaganda which had been so influential in mobilizing the Axis populations during the Second World War, which reached their most extreme manifestation in Germany's perpetration of the Final Solution. Asch wanted to examine how people might resist such malignant pressure.

Asch's experiment involved a "line discrimination task," essentially telling the tester which two lines shown to the group were of equal length. Eight subjects were put in a room together, but only one of the subjects was unaware the test was fixed. The other seven had agreed ahead of time to frequently answer incorrectly, even though the correct answer was obvious.

Only about a quarter of the unaware test subjects consistently resisted the peer pressure to answer incorrectly, although many were clearly conflicted when answering. Interestingly, resistance rose dramatically when at least one other subject guessed correctly. Having even just one ally is a powerful antidote to the pressures of compliance.

We probably all have had this experience in a group setting where you hold an unpopular opinion. You likely keep it to yourself, but if you have a sense someone else agrees with you, you're much more likely to come forward. It's quite likely that, as social animals, we're wired to resist being ostracized.

The Milgram experiments. About ten years after the Asch experiments, in fact, during the trial of Adolf Eichmann in Jerusalem, Yale psychologist Stanley Milgram conducted further tests on obedience, this time involving the role of authority figures. The study employed adult men from diverse walks of life and with varying levels of education and tasked them to obey an authority figure who instructed them to perform acts conflicting with their personal conscience. Participants were led to believe that they were taking part in an experiment on learning, and how pain affects our ability to retain information. The pain came in the form of electric shocks administered to a "student." These (fake) shocks would increase with each error made by the student until they reached fatal levels.

Milgram invited fellow psychologists to predict the outcome. Most believed that only a tiny fraction of the participants would fully obey the instructions. They were wrong. Compliance was high and was heightened when the authority figure assumed responsibility for the consequences of the "shocks."

The outcome of the experiments scared Milgram himself: "The results as I observe them in the laboratory, are disturbing," he said in the closing narration to a documentary version of his test. "They raised the possibility that human nature cannot be counted on to insulate men from brutality and inhumane treatment at the direction of malevolent authority. A substantial proportion of people do what they are told to do irrespective of the content of the act and without limitations of conscience, so long as they perceive that the command comes from a legitimate authority.

"If in this study an anonymous experimenter could successfully command adults to subdue a 50-year-old man and force on him painful electric shocks against his protests," continued Milgram, "one can only wonder what government, with its vastly greater authority and prestige, can command of its subjects."

Importantly, not all participants obeyed the experimenter's demands, and Milgram's studies shed light on the factors that enable people to stand up to authority. In fact, as sociologist Matthew Hollander has written, we may be able to learn from the participants who disobeyed, as their strategies may enable us to respond more effectively to an unethical situation. The Milgram experiment suggests that human beings are susceptible to authority, but it also demonstrates that obedience is not inevitable.

The analysis of Eichmann on trial, coupled with the lessons drawn from iconic psychology experiments, should give all of us pause to consider the consequences of groupthink, of using the collective approval or disapproval of a population for both justification and motivation. Crowds can be wrong. Crowds can be malevolent. Eccentrics and outliers may be insightful. Ideas and policies must stand on their own merits.

These past couple of years have been one massive COVID test, and by that I don't mean anything strictly scientific. It has been a test of our social sensibilities, our tendencies towards both cohesion and ostracization, and above all a test of our morality. I think what it's revealed is that we are so much more inclined to sliding scales and double standards than we ever would have thought, or at least cared to admit. There has been a near-complete collapse of the concept that was a hallmark of twentieth-century social progress: *my body, my rights.*

The erasure of individualism that's behind the collapse seems on the surface to enhance the possibility of unity. But unity can exist in more than one form, and the unity found at the end of a bayonet point or government edict is no stronger (I would hope less, in fact) than the unity that comes from the respect for the uniqueness of each member of the body politic and a sharing of common values and purposes.

Yes, it's a given that democracy does require a certain kind of cooperation. It requires individuals not just to think of themselves and for themselves, but to think about how their actions will affect their neighbours. I like to envision a solid democracy as a talented and seasoned choir. Not every person needs to sing exactly the same part in exactly the same way with exactly the same pitch in order for it to work. In fact, beauty comes from a kind of harmonic discord.

You can have a unity with discord built into the system. You can allow for diversity and disagreement and a multiplicity of religious views and moral views, and different vocations and different ways of raising your family. You can allow for that in a democracy, and if we slide into the view where we expect people to live exactly the same way, believe exactly the same things, we have lost something of tremendous value.

Another great philosopher of the Enlightenment wrote eloquently about the dangers of such a loss. Immanuel Kant, writing a century after Hobbes' remedy for the "nasty, brutish and short" lives of his contemporaries, saw freedom as central to an enlightened world:

> This enlightenment requires nothing but freedom—and the most innocent of all that may be called 'freedom': freedom to make public use of one's reason in all matters. Now I hear the cry from all sides: 'Do not argue!' The officer says: 'Do not argue—drill!' The tax collector: 'Do not argue—pay!' The pastor: 'Do not argue—believe!' Only one ruler in the world says: 'Argue as much as you please, but obey!' We find restrictions on freedom everywhere. But which restriction is harmful to enlightenment? Which restriction is innocent, and which advances enlightenment? I reply: the public use of one's reason must be free at all times, and this alone can bring enlightenment to mankind."

CHAPTER 6

DO NOT GO GENTLY

After a speech I gave recently, a man from the audience approached me for a conversation. "I heard everything you have to say," he said. "I agree with you, but what should I do tomorrow?"

It was a good question, a perfect question, in fact. I should have expected it. Instead, I just looked at him and answered, "I'm not sure. I don't know what the most effective thing an individual person can do to achieve all these more general things I'm talking about."

We've talked about untethering from the academy, about the banality of evil and the perils of conformity, about the Socratic demand to live an examined life. But what about the little guy who lives on Maple Street and works at the convenience store? What *is* he supposed to do tomorrow?

At the time I answered, I truly didn't know. I've learned a lot in the ensuing weeks, and I still don't have all the answers. But I do have a strategy to find some of them.

Let's first pause and take stock of where we're at. How are we doing personally, and as a society at large? How are the anti-COVID measures, the vaccine rollout (now in its booster phase), and the masking edicts and the lockdowns going? How does all this square with our expectations for freedom?

I asked another audience to do that reckoning with me. Yes, it's a self-selected group that wouldn't pass official polling muster, but I asked anyway: "How many of you felt freer two years ago?" All hands went up. "Ten years ago?" Hardly anyone lowered a hand. Apart from the raw COVID statistics, it is clear many people are not doing well in terms of their sense of freedom and belonging.

There is an obvious retort, one that's been made to me in person and certainly through social media: of course our freedoms are curtailed, *we're fighting an existential war* and sacrifices must be made!

But is that the case? Is COVID-19 an existential threat? The numbers tell a different story, whether it's the virus' lethality or the heavily skewed age groups most at risk. The science I look at shows clearly that we would have been out of this thing in 2020 if we had just circled the health wagons around the most vulnerable in our population and let life go on far closer to normal for the rest of us.

On the other side of the ledger, I think we're losing a lot. We've lost a lot. We're accepting and entrenching some very restrictive, non-democratic principles in the service of the idea that we're enmeshed in an emergency. And as long as we feel so hamstrung, we won't have the freedom to look at the situation carefully and objectively.

Which leads to my first piece of advice: take a step back. The moment you finish this book, get some distance from the "madding crowd" and find your own space where you have the freedom to get a grasp of your thoughts and your perspective. Stop drinking from the firehose of daily COVID-19 updates, nudge messages, social media bun fights, cable TV pundit wars. Shut off the noise so we can allow thoughts to emerge from the silence. Those are more likely to be our own, coming from within, rather than the echoes from outside.

If those thoughts don't appear right away, don't despair. At least you've bought yourself a measure of peace and quiet, rare commodities at this point in the twenty-first century.

Second, once we've gathered our composure and have a better sense of our own understanding of the situation, we can start to approach other people with the goal of rebuilding our ability to communicate respectfully and productively. What will this look like? What would it require of us? It could happen at your family dinner table, or in the lineup waiting for your double-double, or chatting with a fellow parent as you pick your kid up from school, or engaging with the Uber driver on the way to an appointment.

Have a conversation where the primary currency isn't argumentative victory. Listen to understand the other person, and not just to hear when there's a gap that allows you to jump in and score a point. Make room for questions that aren't rhetorical or designed to trap the other person in a logical gotcha. Ask to find out what and how others think. Imagine if our first thought in approaching others was to glean thoughts from them and not just download our own thoughts on them. What if we tried hard to make it very clear to others that we want to hear what they think and why they think it, that we value their opinions?

I think Toronto city councillor Kristyn Wong-Tam nailed it when she made a plea recently for discourse over divide. "Being Canadian does not mean we are all exactly the same," she wrote in a *Toronto Sun* op-ed. "Our friends and family who have made different decisions from us are not second-class social pariahs, but people who have been thoughtful in arriving at their own individual health decisions and we must respect that." (Sadly, two days later she felt compelled to respond on Twitter to an all-too-predictable social media outcry stemming from her plea for discourse: "I wanted to talk about how we can continue to build trust across different and diverse communities. I was sharing my perspective and lived experience and was not offering any medical advice. I'm truly sorry this caused any confusion or upset.") In the aftermath of her column, which generated considerable social media blowback, Wong-Tam felt compelled to apologize for her remarks. Just days later, she announced she won't seek to extend her position as vice-chair of the Toronto Board of Health.

Finding common ground is critical. Remember the Asch experiments on conformity from the previous chapter? One of their more fascinating revelations was the importance of finding an ally in the group. When even one other person made judgments that agreed with the test subject, he was much more likely to stick to his original assessment than go along with the (deliberately incorrect) crowd. Just one person can make a massive difference when it comes to breaking free of a coercive (deliberate or otherwise) environment.

When it comes to a coercive environment, I've noticed something about many of the people who have spoken out about Canada's approach to handling COVID. More than a few grew up in eastern Europe, behind the Iron Curtain during the Cold War, in South Africa in the wake of apartheid, or who are only a generation away from those experiences and have learned about them from family.

They are eager to tell me, sometimes with a shaky voice and tears in their eyes, that Canadians don't understand the perilous path we're on. Because we haven't experienced it, but they have lived it, sometimes with grave consequences. They'll say it straight to me, a third-generation Canadian born into security and comfort, "you can't understand this because you've never faced this, you haven't seen the early signs of it." I can feel chills as I'm saying it right now. Because for them it's so clear that these initial steps encroach on freedoms they see as hard won, and the price of sacrifice is too high given the manageable threat in front of us.

But they do have hope that we can veer away from our current dangerous course. It's a hope founded in their own history: the places they came from did, in fact, change course in rather dramatic fashion. It's still a marvel to me to think that in less time than my daughter has been alive, hundreds of millions of people shrugged off the chains of totalitarianism that had bound them for decades and did so with very little bloodshed (normally the calling card for change in the twentieth century). So, they have a hope that we'll work this out, a hope founded on their own life experiences.

Hope is something I've been thinking about a lot of late. How much we need hope, why so many appear to have lost hope, and whether hope itself is a civic virtue in our twenty-first-century democracy.

By *civic virtue,* I mean something like a character trait or habit of thought or action that is essential for democracy to flourish, perhaps even function. And if it is important for democracy, then it is something that must be developed in, and exhibited by, its citizens if we are to survive and, yes, flourish. And while we may not need hope (or at least think that we do) as much when we are doing well, hope is a key civic virtue when democracy faces significant challenges, such as war, an economic crisis, social strife, or a global pandemic.

American philosopher Nancy Snow wrote about "resilience and hope as a democratic civic virtue" in the anthology *Virtues in the Public Sphere*, where she claims that, by definition, hope as a democratic civic virtue requires openness. It follows that we need to approach each other with a similar openness, a curiosity and genuine interest in what we all contribute to society. Back to my "listen" edict, right?

Much of Snow's inspiration is drawn from the works of Walt Whitman, especially his works "Song of Myself" and *Democratic*

Vistas. Both touch on the theme of hope as a democratic civic virtue. But what is particularly interesting to me about Whitman's comments, and especially relevant for the crisis we face, is his idea that poetry and literature can help to build hope and shape the national character in ways that wouldn't seem obvious to those of us caught up in the hurly burly of argument and social combat. Many of us have lost literature (and our arts, more generally) as a key facet of life, so it isn't surprising at all to me that we face democratic deterioration as well.

Much of Whitman's initial impetus was to analyze the problems of life in America in the nineteenth century. But his advice would serve us well today. He calls for an ennobling national body of literature as the way to cultivate the kind of character and ideals necessary to support a flourishing democracy. Literature, Whitman wrote, "has become the only general means of morally influencing the world," its enduring, archetypes and characters help shape the virtues and political ideals of future states. Long after the governments and social structures of ancient Greece and Rome (indeed all great and vanished civilizations) have crumbled, what remains? Their literature, their art, their philosophy, their ideals.

In *Democratic Vistas*, Whitman wrote, "the literature, songs, esthetics, etc., of a country are of importance principally because they furnish the materials and suggestions of personality for the women and men of that country, and enforce them in a thousand effective ways." He continued with this theme: "Did you, too, O friend, suppose democracy was only for elections, for politics, and for a party name? I say democracy is only of use there that it may pass on and come to its flower and fruits in manners, in the highest forms of interaction between men, and their beliefs—in religion, literature, colleges, and schools—democracy in all public and private life."

While Whitman writes as an unapologetic American, I think his viewpoint is entirely relevant for the problems we face today. The fact that literature and the arts "furnish the materials and suggestions of personality . . . and enforce them in a thousand effective ways" is, at least in part, why a comprehensive liberal arts education is so important, and why we have lost much in our attempt to over-specialize and create "experts" with a very narrow range of expertise.

Hope should be the foundation of resilience, which has rarely been more important in our recent history. How well a society endures a crisis or rebounds from one would seem to say a lot about how strong it was when it entered the crisis.

But resilience, almost by definition, requires flexibility and malleability. Like the building stone "brownstone" (also known as "freestone" for its ability to be cut in any direction), being adaptable and even malleable prepare us to weather life's storms. If so, how are we to achieve such resilience? Ours is increasingly a culture that has grown ossified. Uniformity of thought is a growing presence even off campus, with coercion pushed through social media or the heavy hand of government. We are not faring well in the current crisis. Wouldn't we be more likely to weather a crisis well, and to recover from it, if we had more flexibility and more resilience? And aren't we made largely through embracing qualities like tolerance, understanding, and true diversity?

Moving forward, it seems to me that we need to think hard about the civic and moral virtues we've lost. The commitments of citizens to the democratic project can't simply be taken for granted. We aren't all equally good at it and we certainly aren't born with the virtues democracy requires. It demands work to get along with others and a special kind of work to understand how we have strayed from a good path and how we might find our way back.

Some common human emotions—fear, shame, and envy come to mind—are the enemies of our feelings of compassion and empathy towards our fellow citizens. Fear makes it difficult to think about anything else but oneself (and, specifically, the immediate things that threaten us) and our immediate circle. Envy enhances hostility. And when one group, the dominant group, presents its way of life as normal and morally superior, it can successfully shame and stigmatize the ways of others as shameful, unworthy, destructive, selfish, and undemocratic. We see this every day in social media and it has started to percolate through to everyday life.

Even when we disagree, we need to be gracious towards each other, indeed much more gracious than we are being now. I think grace helps us to employ a principle of charity when we approach each other. It also opens the possibility of curiosity which, as mentioned, requires empathy or a presumption that there might be some value in another person's thoughts, that their value doesn't just consist in being a cog in the larger collectivist machine or an ally in our war.

As for the virtues we'll need moving forward, let's also realize that some of the measures we've taken over the past two years have lessened our capacity to experience the emotions necessary for virtue.

Masking, one of the great virtue signals of the pandemic, is one example. Virtue signalling is the attempt to demonstrate to others your right action or good character by expressing certain opinions or engaging in actions that will be acceptable to them. Wearing a mask—the right kind of mask, in the right way, in the right places and for the right activities and people—signifies a commitment to a certain view of public health and to the dominant narrative of this moment in history. But it isn't without its moral costs, costs that may not appear on the balance sheet of a government or public health unit. There are psychological and social costs to masking, making it more than just an immunological and epidemiological issue. For a social species, covering the face hurts in the social dimension, particularly in small children whose brains are acutely tuned to facial and emotional recognition. The distancing that often accompanies masking policies limits our ability to express friendliness and compassion, and to see those things in others. All the pandemic policies that limit and mediate our social interactions with others make it easier to see the other as 'other,' make it harder to feel and express empathy, and to be less acutely aware of our shared humanity.

These measures can all be assassins of hope. They have the potential to undermine the ingredients needed for empathy, compassion and grace. Anything that prevents us from seeing others—literally and figuratively—is an obstacle to be overcome. And we're already tasked with having to overcome so much just to stay on an even keel.

Well, I've veered away from advice meant to uplift and motivate and fallen once again into outlining the darkness we need to penetrate. But I wouldn't have written this book if I thought that was an impossible task.

In many respects, I am an unlikely person to be on the tip of this spear. Although I rarely go with the flow or follow the crowd, I am, at the same time, an unlikely dissenter and an uncharacteristic rebel.

After all, I'm an academic and a relatively mild-mannered and unassuming one at that. More of a thinker and bookworm than a lobbyist and rioter. It's not that I desire to spend my life confined to the metaphorical armchair, but the armchair is a pretty comfortable place. I guess I never thought there would be a need, or that there would be an opportunity, to venture much beyond it.

And to be quite honest, instead of doing interviews, writing and giving speeches, etc., I would rather spend my days enjoying simple moments with my daughter, reading books together, catching ladybugs, playing dress-up. But I also want a world for her in which her books aren't burned, her words aren't censored, and her ideas aren't threatened, coerced, and 'nudged.' And so I continue to do what I do. It's a battle we may not win, but there is value, I think, in the trying.

People often ask, how can you spend so much time doing this? Don't you miss other parts of your life? Indeed, I do. I am missing a great deal. But my feeling is there are seasons to life. And this is the season for doing what I am doing now. This season is also yours.

Are you familiar with *The Life of Pi*? Author Yann Martel talks about the trade-off involved with living in a zoo. In the zoo, you are well fed and have everything you need to live safely and comfortably without constantly fearing for your life, but you are caged; in the wild, you are cold, hungry, and constantly afraid of being someone else's meal. But you are perfectly free. Which would you rather be: fed or free? Is that a choice we need to make or can we build a democracy in which both are possible?

Why does it seem that so many today are choosing the life in the cage? Talking about rights and freedom these days seems to either fall on deaf ears or be dismissed as irrelevant or even selfish. There is a frightening majority in this country that doesn't believe anything that truly matters is being lost. Have we decided that a life of comfort, security and conformity—if that is even possible, or if it comes at the cost of compliance and conformity—is worth the price of freedom? How can you rally a people to stand up for their rights when they don't think their rights are slipping away? What use is there in trying to emancipate someone who doesn't realize she is not truly free? What if you're blind to the cage that has been erected around you? What if you helped to build it?

How do we break out of the cage? How do we regain our sanity and rebuild our democracy? Perhaps it's time to get a bit noisy. Studies have proven that once an idea is adopted by just 10 per cent of the population, it has reached a tipping point where ideas, opinions, and beliefs are likely to be rapidly adopted by the rest. A *noisy* 10 per cent is all it takes.

Democracy, "rule of the people," doesn't just allow for freedom of expression and inquiry; it requires it. But let's acknowledge right now the stiff headwinds we all face while pushing back against the prevailing orthodoxies surrounding our COVID-19 response.

It almost beggars belief that this has to be said, but it does: you are *not* a bad person for demanding evidence, you *are not* a bad person for trusting your instincts, and you are *not* a bad person for wanting to think for yourself. In fact, the opposite is true. If you are worried about a loss of justice, if you are worried about what kinds of lives will be possible for our children, if you want your country back—the country that was once the envy of the world—then now is the time to act. There is no reason to wait, there is no luxury or excuse to wait. We need you now.

Now is the time to call our politicians and message our media. Now is the time to protest, now is the time to challenge and even disobey our government. Now is the time to ask thoughtful questions around the dinner table. Now is the time to hold each other up and not break each other down. As the quotation attributed to anthropologist Margaret Mead goes, "Never doubt that a small group of thoughtful, committed citizens can change the world; indeed, it's the only thing that ever has."

Now is the time to work for Canada to recapture its Enlightenment ideals of freedom and fearless inquiry.

More than two centuries ago, Immanuel Kant (you met him in the last chapter) made a case for humanity to grow up. His take on enlightenment wasn't purely intellectual, it was a plea for us to emerge as a fully adult species.

"Enlightenment is man's emergence from his self-imposed immaturity," he wrote in his 1784 essay "What is Enlightenment?" "Immaturity is the inability to use one's understanding without guidance from another. This immaturity is self-imposed when its cause lies not in lack of understanding, but in lack of resolve and courage to use it without guidance from another. *Sapere Aude!* 'Have courage to use your own understanding!'—that is the motto of enlightenment."

This is so interesting and timely. What Kant is calling for is exactly what we need now. When I tell audiences that we are in a "pandemic of compliance," it's not so much that we lack knowledge or even understanding, but that we lack the resolve or intention or maybe even just the courage to use our knowledge without guidance from another. In an epistle addressed to his friend Lollius, Horace offers a fable in which a fool waits for a stream to cease flowing before attempting to cross while the wise man forgoes comfort and attempts to cross anyway. Horace advocates not only effort in overcoming life's obstacles but courage in seeking understanding for oneself.

Sapere aude! Dare to know, dare to be wise. Find the courage to use your own understanding. Kant tells us that not only do we need to use reason publicly in order to be enlightened, but we must not think that freedom to use our own reason is dangerous. If Kant is right, it seems that we first need the freedom to use our own reason in order to have an enlightenment; freedom to reason for oneself is not the product of the enlightenment, but its prerequisite.

Find the courage to see that we are not each other's enemies, and we are not alone in our drive to change circumstances for the better. We don't need to comply or agree about everything to have a healthy democracy. In fact, a compliant and monochromatic populace is a sign of an ailing democracy with a dim future. A choir in which everyone sings the same part is never as beautiful as the one in which people sing different and complementary parts; the beauty and unity in that harmony are unmatchable.

A society in which we respect each other's differences is a true democracy. And that democracy is just beyond our fingertips. We just have to want it, and reach out and grab it. So let's cross our arms in defiance. Speak up. Refuse to comply. Ask questions. Dismantle the cage. Cross the stream while it is still flowing.

Choose courage. *Sapere aude*!

APPENDIX 1

As 2021 draws to a close, there are almost daily reports of people losing positions or otherwise suffering for their principled opposition to COVID-19 measures. While hardly comprehensive, the following list gives a sense of the integrity and the diversity of these individuals:

Corporal Daniel Bulford

RCMP Corporal Daniel Bulford left his job as a sniper on the security detail of Prime Minister Justin Trudeau on November 2. He had been off work since October, when the federal government announced that all public employees would have to be vaccinated to stay on their jobs.

Bulford isn't quite forty-years-old and in top shape. In a recent interview he said, "it appears that someone like myself . . . (is) likely at greater risk of an adverse event from one of the vaccines than we are of severe illness or disease from coronavirus."

He also acts as a spokesperson for Mounties for Freedom, a group of fellow officers that formed in 2021 to push back against the RCMP's implementation of mandatory vaccination. The group states it is "against the forced and coerced medical intervention of Canadians and against the discrimination faced by those who have exercised their right to decide on their bodily autonomy."

Dr. Francis Christian

Dr. Francis Christian, a surgeon and professor at the University of Saskatchewan in Saskatoon, lost his job with the university after questioning the need for COVID-19 vaccinations for children and challenging the concept of informed consent as it has been applied in the province.

Christian has practiced medicine for more than twenty years and was appointed director of the surgical humanities program and director of quality and patient safety in 2018 (he also co-founded the surgical humanities program). He edits the *Journal of The Surgical Humanities*.

In June 2021, Dr. Christian sent a written statement to more than two hundred of his colleagues outlining his concerns. He prefaced it by saying he was pro-vaccine. "The principle of informed consent is being consistently violated in this province for the m-RNA vaccine for our kids," he wrote. "I have not met a single vaccinated child or parent who has been adequately informed and who then understand the risks of this vaccine or its benefits." Shortly after the statement's release the Saskatchewan Health Authority ended its contract with Christian and the university suspended him pending a review of his actions and statements.

Dr. Rochagné Kilian

Dr. Rochagné Kilian, a specialist in family and emergency medicine, was suspended in October 2021 by the College of Physicians and Surgeons of Ontario. Kilian has been a visible and outspoken critic of the pandemic response, including vaccine safety, and mandates, and lockdown measures.

Kilian's licence was originally restricted in mid-October (she was barred from issuing exemptions for vaccinations, masking, and testing) after the college determined her conduct "exposes or is likely to expose patients to harm or injury." Two weeks later the restriction was broadened to a full suspension.

In August, she quit as an emergency doctor with Grey Bruce

Health Services, which operates five hospitals in south-central Ontario, to protest the imminent implementation of vaccination mandates. "For eighteen months I've been living through this whole pandemic," she said. "I was on the front lines, literally on the front lines as an ER physician from the start, and I could no longer remain silent."

Rick Nicholls

The member of provincial parliament for the Ontario riding of Chatham-Kent-Leamington, Rick Nicholls' battle against COVID vaccine mandates ended with his exile from the Progressive Conservative party caucus and his removal as deputy speaker of the legislature, a position he had held for seven years.

Nicholls refused the legislature's vaccination mandate for personal reasons. "I took the premier at his word that vaccination is a choice and that all Ontarians have a constitutional right to make such a choice," Nicholls said at the time of his caucus expulsion in August 2021. "Like almost two million eligible Ontarians, I choose to exercise this autonomy over my own body while continuing to work hard for the people of Ontario."

Now sitting as an independent, Nicholls announced in October that he won't seek re-election, effecting ending his provincial political career.

John Rakich

John Rakich has worked at General Motors in St. Catharines, Ont. for close to forty years, and was an active member of his union (now Unifor) for most of that time. His pushback against vaccine mandates ended that.

In August 2021, the union asked Rakich about his vaccination status before he was set to help out another local in Ontario. He refused to say, out of privacy considerations, and was told by Unifor to stand down from helping.

A few weeks later, when vaccine mandates were announced, Rakich again refused to confirm his status. That led to a confrontation directly with Unifor's national president Jerry Dias, who told Rakich the privacy statutes he was citing didn't apply under COVID. He was terminated from his union role.

"We are not anti-vaxx people," Rakich said in a recent interview. "There are actually a lot of vaccinated people who are taking the position that we're taking, and are willing to lose their jobs, believe it or not, because they don't believe in the mandates, they don't believe in people being forced to take a medical procedure against their will."

APPENDIX 2

Dr. Julie Ponesse co-authored the following letter on behalf of the Canadian COVID Care Alliance, to the *Toronto Star* following the publication of its incendiary August 26, 2021 front page that purported to examine the polarized debate over COVID vaccinations.

The bulk of the page was taken up by a collection of tweets in very large type, all of the same tenor. Here is a selection:

"If an unvaccinated person catches it from someone who is vaccinated, boohoo, too bad."

"I have no empathy left for the wilfully unvaccinated. Let them die."

"Unvaccinated patients do not deserve ICU beds."

"At this point, who cares. Stick the unvaccinated in a tent outside and tend to them when the staff has time."

Two days later the *Star*'s public editor, Bruce Campion-Smith, addressed the considerable public outcry. His apology, in my eyes, wasn't nearly strong enough:

Campion-Smith noted the tweets as presented offered "virtually no context." Even those who grasped the context, he added, noted "the selected tweets presented just one side of this debate" and were upset the country's largest-circulation newspaper would put such hurtful comments on the front page.

"The *Star* wound up stoking the very divisions it sought to write about."

Our letter:

Hatred towards the unvaccinated is a result of continuing misinformation in the media about what COVID-19 vaccines can and cannot achieve.

The August 26 *Toronto Star* front page was a disgrace to a newspaper that is proud of its inclusivity and investigative reporting. The half-hearted apology by the *Star's* public editor two days later was a step in the right direction. Yet, it did not address the core of the issue.

The public's misconception of the COVID-19 vaccines, reflected in the hateful front-page messages, is based on a misunderstanding of the function of these vaccines. A mis-understanding that is being perpetuated in the media and by public health officials and politicians. Unlike many traditional vaccines, the currently available COVID-19 vaccines with their waning efficacy do not provide "sterilizing immunity." This type of vaccine is also called "leaky", because it cannot prevent infection with the target virus. Vaccinated persons can still carry and transmit SARS-CoV-2, just like the unvac-cinated. Instead, the vaccines were developed to protect the recipient from symptomatic COVID-19.

Taking the vaccine is an individual decision, in which each patient, under fully informed consent and without external pressures, weighs the benefits and risks for their own health. Sadly, this fact has been lacking in the deployment and promotion of these vaccines. A person's COVID-19 vaccination may protect them, but does not substantially impact the health of any other person around them. Consequently, asking for someone's vaccination status, or mandating vaccines, is based on flawed logic.

Mandating vaccines for healthy youth and the working-age population is particularly misguided, given the low to non-existing threat of serious COVID-19 and the potential for vaccine injury.

The nature of these vaccines provides no rational basis for restrictions of bodily autonomy, medical privacy, or other civil rights. The vaccines should be reserved for those elderly and vulnerable individuals who choose to take them.

Supporting hate messaging against those who choose not to be vaccinated is not only undemocratic but it fuels the flames of betrayal, contempt, and severe moral injury between citizens. The *Toronto Star* has worked hard to transcend these moral failings in the past and we respectfully request a prominent, front-page letter of apology to redress them now.

> *Drs. Steven Pelech, Julie Ponesse, and Claus Rinner*
> *on behalf of the Canadian Covid Care Alliance.*